NEUROSCIENCE RESEARCH PROGRESS

NEUROPATHIC PAIN

RISK FACTORS, TYPES AND MANAGEMENT STRATEGIES

NEUROSCIENCE RESEARCH PROGRESS

Additional books in this series can be found on Nova's website under the Series tab.

Additional e-books in this series can be found on Nova's website under the e-book tab.

NEUROSCIENCE RESEARCH PROGRESS

NEUROPATHIC PAIN

RISK FACTORS, TYPES AND MANAGEMENT STRATEGIES

ALYSSA L. RIDER
EDITOR

New York

For permission to use material from this book please contact us:
Telephone 631-231-7269; Fax 631-231-8175
Web Site: http://www.novapublishers.com

Additional color graphics may be available in the e-book version of this book.

Library of Congress Cataloging-in-Publication Data

ISBN: 978-1-63321-963-2

Library of Congress Control Number: 2014949885

Published by Nova Science Publishers, Inc. † New York

Contents

Preface

This book discusses non-invasive brain stimulation to control neuropathic pain. It also discusses neuropathic pain in patients with spinal cord injury and the new management strategies for these individuals.

Chapter 1 – Neuropathic pain (NP) affects large population worldwide determining increased direct and indirect costs and significantly alters the patients' quality of life and psychological morbidity. NP is defined according to the IASP as ‘‘pain caused by a lesion or disease of the somatosensory system’’ although many studies in human and animal models have proved that neuroplastic changes in non-sensory structures may also contribute to NP mechanisms. Moreover, it has been shown that plasticity within the nociceptive and antinociceptive systems may be “maladaptive” contributing essentially to the peripheral and central sensitization of pain, rather than to compensate for the loss of function or to adjust their activity in response to new situations or changes in their environment. However, despite the accumulating knowledge on pathophysiological mechanisms of NP the pharmacological treatment is mainly symptom-oriented, with satisfactory pain relief in less than 50% of patients. Therefore, NP management should be performed by a multidisciplinary team that needs to move from a simply suppression of symptoms to a combination of pharmacological treatment with techniques of prevention and correction of maladaptive plasticity. Among the non-invasive brain stimulation techniques, there is accumulating evidence that the repetitive transcranial magnetic stimulation (rTMS) as well as the transcranial direct current stimulation (tDCS) can produce analgesic effects in subjects with NP conditions of various etiologies, including in those showing resistance to conventional therapies. Whereas tDCS alters spontaneous neuronal excitability in a polarity-specific manner in targeted cortical regions, rTMS mechanisms are based on electromagnetic induction to generate electric currents in the brain. In general, low-frequency (0.2-1Hz) rTMS and cathodal tDCS decrease, and high-frequency (5-25Hz) rTMS and anodal tDCS enhance the excitability of neurons of the targeted cortical areas. However, only high frequency-rTMS and anodal tDCS promote synaptic plasticity and have been proved to be effective in alleviating NP. Although their exact underlying neurobiologic mechanisms of pain modulation remain poorly understood many research suggests that rTMS and tDSC induced analgesia following motor cortex or dorsolateral prefrontal cortex stimulation is probably mediated through functional changes in the activity of several cerebral areas such as the thalamus, the anterior cingulate, insular, and prefrontal cortices involved in modulation of the sensory, emotional and cognitive components of pain. Furthermore, the long lasting antalgic effect following multiple sessions of rTMS or tDCS as well as their cumulative and synergistic benefits when combined with behavioral treatments make these non-invasive stimulation techniques of significant clinical relevance as adjuvant therapy of NP and pain-related affective and cognitive comorbidities.

Chapter 2 – Pain is a common complication in patients following spinal cord injury (SCI), with studies demonstrating up to 80% of patients reporting some form of pain in the years after their injury. Pain can be divided into multiple different subtypes including nociceptive, neuropathic, and psychogenic. Neuropathic pain, and more specifically central neuropathic pain, makes up a substantial percentage of all pain symptoms in patients with SCI. Given the high prevalence of central neuropathic pain in patients with SCI, proper identification and treatment is imperative. Indeed, identification of pain subtypes is a vital step toward determining appropriate treatment, and once determined, a variety of treatment measures can be undertaken. Medications commonly utilized to treat neuropathic pain include anticonvulsants, tricyclic antidepressants, antispastic agents, and opioids. Non-pharmacologic treatment strategies include spinal cord stimulation, physical therapy, physical modalities, psychological interventions, and acupuncture. Additionally, intrathecal delivery of certain medications have become increasingly popular and been shown to significantly reduce neuropathic pain, while causing fewer systemic side effects than oral drugs in patients with SCI. Despite all of the available treatment options and ongoing advances in the field of SCI medicine, providing adequate treatment of central neuropathic pain after SCI continues to be challenging. Management of central neuropathic pain, as with other forms of chronic pain, is complex and often requires a multifaceted and integrative approach. It is therefore extremely important for clinicians to have a good understanding of how central neuropathic pain arises, as well all the available and appropriate treatment options for patients displaying this sort of pain.

In this chapter the author will discuss the pathophysiology, identification, and treatment options for patients with SCI displaying central neuropathic pain, giving recommendations where appropriate. The author hope that this will not only provide a better understanding of central neuropathic pain for physicians in various subspecialties, but that it will also help guide future research on this important subject.

Chapter 3 – Traumatic spinal cord injury (SCI) results in loss of motor, sensory and autonomic functions below the site of injury. About two-thirds of SCI patients develop central neuropathic pain that interferes with daily functioning and ability to participate in life activities, reducing their quality of life. Neuropathic pain following SCI is caused by several physio-pathological events that include: (i) disruption of blood vessels associated with hemorrhage, hypoxia, hypoglycemia, and infiltration of neutrophils, monocytes and T-lymphocytes, (ii) necrosis of neurons, glial cells and endothelial cells with the release of potassium ions and glutamate, and (iii) release of cytokines, proteases, prostaglandins and free radicals by infiltrated blood cells and re-activated microglia and astrocytes. All these factors that appeared in the lesion site are able to stimulate nociceptive-specific and wide -dynamic range nociceptive neurons located in the dorsal horn of adjacent spinal cord segments, causing excitation of the anterolateral spinal cord pathway and pain. In addition, these factors also induce central sensitization of nociceptive neurons, and activation of several intracellular signaling pathways that produce genetic and phenotypic changes of nociceptive spinal neurons. These "new" neurons are able to respond more easily to afferent peripheral inputs but also to central pro-inflammatory agents. Then, subjects develop neuropathic pain, including hyperalgesia and allodynia. These types of pain are consuming, chronic and largely refractory to treatment. Thus, new pharmacological treatments or strategies should be developed for reducing neuropathic pain in SCI subjects. The knowledge of the new activated signaling pathways in nociceptive spinal cord neurons after SCI may be crucial for designing novel pharmacological treatments. This chapter gives an overview of the pathological events observed in SCI subjects that develop neuropathic pain, the main intracellular pathways activated in nociceptive neurons during neuropathic pain and new pharmacological approaches focused in phytotherapies such as polyphenols, flavonoids, terpenoids and alkaloids.

In: Neuropathic Pain
Editor: Alyssa L. Rider

ISBN: 978-1-63321-963-2

Chapter 1

Non-Invasive Brain Stimulation to Control Neuropathic Pain

Sergiu Albu[1], Joan Vidal[2,3,4] and Hatice Kumru[2,3,4*]

[1]Clinical Laboratory of Affective Neuroscience of Pain, Department of Psychology, Texas A&M University, College Station, US
[2]Institut Guttmann, Institut Universitari de Neurorehabilitació adscrit a la UAB, 08916 Badalona – Barcelona, Spain.
[3]Univ Autonoma de Barcelona, Bellaterra (Cerdanyola del Vallès), Spain
[4]Fundació Institut d'Investigació en Ciències de la Salut Germans Trias i Pujol, Badalona, Barcelona, Spain

Abstract

Neuropathic pain (NP) affects large population worldwide determining increased direct and indirect costs and significantly alters the patients' quality of life and psychological morbidity. NP is defined according to the IASP as ''pain caused by a lesion or disease of the somatosensory system'' although many studies in human and animal models have proved that neuroplastic changes in non-sensory structures

* Corresponding author: Hatice Kumru, MD, PhD. Hospital de Neurorehabilitació Institut Guttmann, Camí Can Ruti s/n. Barcelona, 08916 Barcelona, Spain. Tel. + 34 93 497 77 00; Fax +34 93 497 77 15, Email: hkumru@guttmann.com.

may also contribute to NP mechanisms. Moreover, it has been shown that plasticity within the nociceptive and antinociceptive systems may be "maladaptive" contributing essentially to the peripheral and central sensitization of pain, rather than to compensate for the loss of function or to adjust their activity in response to new situations or changes in their environment. However, despite the accumulating knowledge on pathophysiological mechanisms of NP the pharmacological treatment is mainly symptom-oriented, with satisfactory pain relief in less than 50% of patients. Therefore, NP management should be performed by a multidisciplinary team that needs to move from a simply suppression of symptoms to a combination of pharmacological treatment with techniques of prevention and correction of maladaptive plasticity. Among the non-invasive brain stimulation techniques, there is accumulating evidence that the repetitive transcranial magnetic stimulation (rTMS) as well as the transcranial direct current stimulation (tDCS) can produce analgesic effects in subjects with NP conditions of various etiologies, including in those showing resistance to conventional therapies. Whereas tDCS alters spontaneous neuronal excitability in a polarity-specific manner in targeted cortical regions, rTMS mechanisms are based on electromagnetic induction to generate electric currents in the brain. In general, low-frequency (0.2-1Hz) rTMS and cathodal tDCS decrease, and high-frequency (5-25Hz) rTMS and anodal tDCS enhance the excitability of neurons of the targeted cortical areas. However, only high frequency-rTMS and anodal tDCS promote synaptic plasticity and have been proved to be effective in alleviating NP. Although their exact underlying neurobiologic mechanisms of pain modulation remain poorly understood many research suggests that rTMS and tDSC induced analgesia following motor cortex or dorsolateral prefrontal cortex stimulation is probably mediated through functional changes in the activity of several cerebral areas such as the thalamus, the anterior cingulate, insular, and prefrontal cortices involved in modulation of the sensory, emotional and cognitive components of pain. Furthermore, the long lasting antalgic effect following multiple sessions of rTMS or tDCS as well as their cumulative and synergistic benefits when combined with behavioral treatments make these non-invasive stimulation techniques of significant clinical relevance as adjuvant therapy of NP and pain-related affective and cognitive comorbidities.

Neuropathic Pain

Pain is a frequent symptom of neurological disease, and is defined as "an unpleasant sensory and emotional experience associated with actual or potential tissue damage" that has a significant impact on the quality of life, general health status, psychological health, and social and economic wellbeing.

Originally, the term "neuropathic pain" (NP) was used to describe only the "pain causes by a lesion or disease of the peripheral somatosensory nervous system" in painful diabetic neuropathy, neuralgia of trigeminus, post-surgical pain, post-herpetic pain, radicular pain and neurophathic cancer pain whereas central pain was defined as "pain caused by lesion or disease of the central somatosensory nervous system" in stroke, multiple sclerosis and spinal cord injury. Lately, the International Association for the Study of Pain (IASP, 2010) defines NP as ''pain caused by a lesion or disease of the somatosensory system''. These imply that NP can arise from a lesion affecting either the peripheral or the central nervous system.

The prevalence of the NP is highly variable ranging from 3.3% to 8.2% in different populations (Haanpaa et al., 2011). However, most of the studies included chronic pain states associated with multiple conditions and the use of different screening tools may also interfered with the appropiate prevalence estimation. NP also varies across different conditions. Peripheral neuropathy affects about 30% of people with diabetes mellitus and about 16-26% of those patients experience chronic pain (Jensen et al., 2006). Herpes zoster strikes are estimated at 800,000 cases each year in the U.S., most of whom are elderly or immunosuppressed and between 25% and 50% of adults older than 50 years develop postherpetic neuralgia at 3 months after rash onset (Schmader, 2002). Also, a large proportion of persistent post-surgery pain is classified as NP and estimates to range betwee 10% and 50% in prevalence with severe forms in up to 10% of this subgroup of patients (Shipton, 2008).

Data from studies in spinal cord injury (SCI) population estimate that at least 80% of the patients experience pain, one-third of them complaining of intense pain (Calmels et al., 2009). NP is more common in patients with incomplete spinal cord lesions and the severity of pain correlates with elder age at injury and female sex (Norrbrink Budh et al., 2003). Sidall reported that the musculoskeletal pain was the most common type of pain experienced with a general prevalence of 59% in the SCI population. However, the prevalence of NP was also high, with at-level NP in 41% and below-level NP in 34% of the patients, whereas visceral pain was present in 5% of the subjects (Siddall, 2003).

Chronic pain is often mentioned as one of the most important factors affecting the quality of life and psychological well-being after a physical disability, and significantly affects the coping and adaptation after SCI (Soler,

2007). Evidence suggests that people with NP have poorer physical and mental health than those with other types of pain, even when adjusted for pain intensity. The discrepancy between the intensity of pain and quality of life implies that other factors beyond recognition are important for patients with NP and that these factors may influence their activities (NICE, 2013).

Pathophysiological Mechanisms of Neuropathic Pain

Different pathophysiological mechanisms underlying NP in both central nervous system and peripheral nervous system operate together. In some patients, the injury of the nerve causes changes in nociceptive neurons at the molecular level, which become abnormally sensitive and develop a pathological spontaneous activity. Inflammatory reactions occurring on the trunk of the injured nerve can induce ectopic activity of nociceptors, causing spontaneous pain. Hyperactivity in nociceptors induce secondary changes in information processing in neurons in the spinal cord and in the brain. This central sensitization causes input from A-fibers to be perceived as pain (allodynia). Neuroplastic changes in systems of central pain modulation may lead to increased hyperexcitability (Baron, 2009).

In the last decades an increasing number of researches provided evidences that NP states are associated with substantial functional reorganization of cortical and subcortical structures involved in pain processing and endogenous pain modulation, including the primary and secondary somatosensory area, anterior cingulate, orbitofrontal cortex, amygdala, and mesencephalic and pontine reticular formation (deCharms et al., 2005; Lee et al., 2008; Moisset et al., 2011; Moont, 2011; Widerstrom-Noga et al., 2013). Consequently, many non-invasive stimulation techniques have been developed to modulate the activity of these neural structures in order to induce short-term pain relief as well as to promote and strengthen the long-term neuroplastic mechanisms (Nizard et al., 2012).

Neuromodulation for Neuroplasticity to Control Neuropathic Pain

Neuromodulation, defined by the International Neuromodulation Society as a field of science, medicine, and bioengineering that encompasses implantable and non-implantable technologies, electrical or chemical, for the purpose of improving quality of life and functioning of humans (Sakas et al., 2007), also refers to all processes of inhibition, stimulation, modification, regulation or therapeutic alteration of the activity, electrically or chemically, in the central, peripheral or autonomic nervous systems (Sokal andSokal, 2011) whereas neuroplasticity is defined as the ability of the nervous system to respond to intrinsic or extrinsic stimuli by reorganizing its structure, function and connections (Cramer et al., 2011).The neuroplasticity phenomenon is controlled by genetic, epigenetic, and hormonal factors and can be influenced by the morbid states of the individual and the applied therapies. Mechanisms of plasticity leading to stabilization and maintenance of the neuronal circuits or the acquisition of new compensatory mechanisms to the pathological state are considered to be "adaptive" whereas states of excessive, unstable or erroneous plasticity determining loss of function or development of new disorders and symptoms are considered to be "maladaptive" (Cramer et al., 2011). However a state of "metaplasticity" or "plasticity of synaptic plasticity" reflecting the change in the ability to induce subsequent synaptic plasticity (Abraham, 1997) as well as a training-dependent effect of stimulus controllability on future plasticity (Ferguson et al., 2012) opens the possibility for the neuromodulation techniques to control the neuroplasticity mechanism.

Non-Invasive Brain Stimulation

Transcranial magnetic stimulation (TMS) and transcranial direct current stimulation (tDCS) are well known and more commonly used neuromodulation techniques for NP.

Transcranial Magnetic Stimulation

TMS is a non-invasive neurostimulation and neuromodulation technique, based on the principle of electromagnetic induction of an electric field in the discrete brain regions (Rossi et al., 2009). Single TMS pulses can depolarize neurons transiently, but when multiple pulses are applied repetitively- an approach known as repetitive TMS (rTMS)- cortical excitability can be increased or decreased depending on the parameters of stimulation (Pell, 2011). When multiple stimuli of TMS are delivered in trains, one can differentiate ''conventional" and ''patterned" protocols of repetitive stimulation. The term 'fast' or 'high-frequency' rTMS refers to stimulus rates of more than 1 Hz, and the term 'slow' or 'low-frequency' rTMS refers to stimulus rates of 1 Hz or less. Such a classification is based on the different physiological effects and degrees of risk associated with low- and high-frequency rTMS (Rossi et al., 2009). Asynchronous trains, such as theta burst stimulation (TBS) paradigms, refer to rTMS protocols where pulses are applied in bursts of three, delivered at a frequency of 50 Hz and an inter-burst interval of 200 ms (5 Hz) (Oberman et al., 2012). These parameters were originally developed based on studies in both the rodent and human brain indicating that theta rhythms are associated with long term depression (LTD) and long term potentiation (LTP) mechanisms (Di Lazzaro et al., 2011; Pell, 2011).

Mechanisms of Action Underlying the Effects of rTMS and TBS

rTMS can induce changes in cortical excitability at the site of stimulation and transsynaptically at distant sites, which can last for minutes or even hours. Generally is accepted that high frequency rTMS (>1 Hz) increases cortical excitability, whereas low frequencyrTMS (≤1 Hz) decreases cortical excitability (Maeda et al., 2000; Pascual-Leone et al., 1998; Speer et al., 2000) but opposite effects have also been described (Lang et al., 2004; Rothkegel, 2010; Siebner, 2004; Sommer, 2013). Indeed, although the frequency of stimulation has always been considered as the main determinant of the course of neuromodulation the effect of rTMS on neuronal excitability shows a considerable degree of variability across different sessions and subjects as a result of interactions between several stimulation parameters. Aside from the frequency of stimulation these parameters include the geometry of the TMS coil, pulse characteristics such as intensity, shape (monophasic or biphasic) and orientation of the induced current flow, as well as the cortical anatomy and function of the stimulated brain area, the level of cortical inhibition at baseline, the gender and age of the subjects, previous pharmaceutical agents administration, hormonal state and other factors (Pell, 2011).

With different stimulation durations, high frequency rTMS can produce different patterns of long-lasting changes in corticospinal and intracortical excitability in stimulated and unstimulated brain areas. Long-duration (5s) 10Hz subthreshold rTMS produces a long-lasting, consistent suppression of corticospinal excitability and intracortical excitability in both stimulated and unstimulated motor cortex as a function of the stimulation duration, whereas short-duration (1.5s) 10Hz subthresholdrTMS enhances the corticospinal excitability in the stimulated cortex (Jung et al., 2008). This opposite modulatory effects following rTMS with two different stimulation durations are explained by the neurophysiological mechanism underlying TBS. Human studies using single trains of TBS suggest that TBS produces a mixture of facilitatory and inhibitory effects on synaptic transmission, with facilitation building up faster than inhibition. A short, intermittent TBS would favor rapid build-up of facilitation. By contrast, a longer lasting continuous protocol such as continuous TBS would initially produce facilitation, but eventually this would saturate, and inhibitory effects would dominate (Huang et al., 2005).

rTMS or TBS appear to lead to sustained changes in cortical activity lasting well beyond the duration of the TMS application. Lasting inhibitory after-effects of low frequency rTMS and continuous TBS and facilitatory after-effects following high frequency rTMS and intermittent TBS were found on motor corticospinal output in healthy subjects. Various mechanisms have been considered, including synaptic changes resembling LTD and LTP mechanisms, as well as shifts in network excitability, activation of feedback loops, activity-dependent metaplasticity, etc. (Rossi et al., 2009). However, given the NMDA receptors activity dependence of the effects most probable the after-effects is mediated by LTP-like synaptic plasticity (Oberman et al., 2012).

Repetitive TMS over Motor Cortex for Neuropathic Pain

Multiple research have studied the efficacy of different stimulation sites such as the primary motor cortex (M1) and supplementrary motor area, the dorsolateral prefrontal cortex (DLPFC) and the primary somatosensory cortex (S1) on NP. However, the most studied target of rTMS for pain control is the M1. Considering the therapeutic efects of the epidural motor cortex stimulation as a treatment for chronic, refractory NP secondary to central deafferentation reported more than three decades ago (Tsubokawa et al., 1991). Migita and colleagues (1995) provided the first description of rTMS over the M1 as a useful tool to estimate the effectiveness of electrical motor cortex stimulation (Migita et al., 1995). Tsubokawa et al. (1993) reported that when a good pain inhibition was achieved in 11 patients with thalamic pain following electrical premotor cortex stimulation patients reported a slight tingling or mild vibration sensation during stimulation projected in the same area of distribution as their pain. Therefore, the authors suggested that premotor cortex stimulation selectively activated non-nociceptive neurons in the sensory cortex which may be able to inhibit deafferented nociceptive neurons within the cortex. This hypothesis led to other researches looking at rTMS stimulation of the adjacent cortical areas as an alternative to the electrical M1 stimulation. Subsequently, a randomized sham control study in 20 patients with intractable deafferentation pain receiving ten trains of 10-s 5Hz TMS pulses, with 50-s inter train intervals of the M1, the S1, premotor or supplementary motor area showed that 50% of the patients indicated that stimulation of M1, but not other areas, provided significant and beneficial pain relief lasting for 3 hours in spite of the fact that M1, S1, premotor and suplimentary motor cortex areas are located adjacently (Hirayama et al., 2006). However, since the spread of cortical excitability following rTMS over the M1 has been proved to depend on the intensity and frequency of the stimuli (Pascual-Leone et al., 1993), future studies compared the therapeutical effects of different protocols of rTMS over the M1 in pain patients. A single 25 min sessions of focal rTMS (1 Hz, 20 Hz and sham) in a group of patients with chronic central and peripheral NP revealed that immediately after the stimulating session, pain scores were equally decreased by all rTMS modalities (Andre-Obadia et al., 2006). However, the repeated evaluation during the following week showed that 1Hz stimulation provided significantly less analgesia than 20 Hz and placebo, and was pro-algesic in some patients (Andre-Obadia et al., 2006) suggesting that a single session of rTMS can induce not only neuromodulation effects that outlast the duration of the stimulation itself low frequency (off-line effects) but also might determine late modulation effects which can be unmask by repeated measures. Similarly, subthreshold 10Hz rTMS applied to the M1 failed to reduce the pain intensity in a mixed group of patients with chronic, drug-resistant NP (central and peripheral) but significant improvement in thermal sensory perception has been observed (Lefaucheur et al., 2008) which might be relevant for the treatment of thermal allodynia. One of the limitations in these studies was the inclusion of subjects with central and peripheral NP of various neurologic origins sharing the same symptom (pain), but with several independent pathophysiological mechanisms which can be crucial for pain modulation. Threfore, a more rigorous selection of the patients were expected to reveal more prominent pain modulation. Indeed, a single session of 5 Hz rTMS over M1 corresponding to the painful side in 21 patients with central post stroke NP determines a variable effect of pain modulation with >30% pain reduction in about one third of subjects (Hosomi et al., 2013a) but only in a quarter (4 subjects) of motor complete or incomplete SCI patients with chronic NP following 10Hz rTMS with more pronounced pain reduction in incomplete SCI (21%) versus complete SCI (3%) (Jette et al., 2013). These studies indicate that patients with brain lesions are more susceptible to develop rTMS induced analgesia.

Table 1. Summary of demographic and clinical characteristics of the subjects with neuropathic pain udergoing rTMS and tDCS

Authors (year)	Subject population	Number of subjects	Age (years)	Disease duration (years)	Duration of pain
rTMS					
Topper et al. (2003)	PLP	2	33.0	NA	14.5 y
Khedr et al. (2004)	TGNP, CPSP	48	51.9		28.5 mo
Hirayama et al. (2006)	CPSP, post-SCI NP, TGNP, PNP	20	56.8	NA	6.4 y
Andre-Obadia et al. (2006)	CPSP, post-SCI NP, PNP	20	54.3	NA	NA
Lefaucheur et al. (2008)	TGNP, NP secondary to BPL, CPSP, post-SCI NP	46	54.2	>1	>1 y
Borckardt et al. (2009)	PNP	4	46.0	NA	10.2 y
Kang et al. (2009)	post-SCI NP	11	54.8	5	>15 mo
Sampson et al. (2011)	post-SCI NP, PLP, CNP, PNP	9	43.1	NA	8.1 y
Matsumura et al (2012)	CPSP	20	63.6	3.2	38.1mo
Lefaucheur et al. (2012)	TGNP, CPSP, post-SCI NP	14	53.8	NA	4.1 y
Jette et al. (2013)	post-SCI NP	16	50.0	7.8	>3 mo
Ohn et al. (2012)	CPSP	22	54.9	NA	21.9 mo
Onesti et al. (2013)	Diabetic neuropathy	23	70.6	NA	NA
Hosomi et al. (2013)a	CPSP	21	59.6	NA	48.1 mo
Hosomi et al. (2013)b	CPSP, post-SCI NP, PNP	52	60.7	NA	>6 mo

Table 1. (Continued)

Authors (year)	Subject population	Number of subjects	Age (years)	Disease duration (years)	Duration of pain
tDCS					
Fregni et al. (2006)	post-SCI NP	17	35.7	3.5	>3 mo
Antal et al. (2010)	TGNP, CPSP, back pain, fibromyalgia	23	57.1	NA	7.4 y
Soler et al. (2010)	post-SCI NP	39	45.0	8.3	>6 mo
Dos Santos et al. (2012)	TGNP	1	62.0	NA	NA
Wrigley et al. (2012)	post-SCI NP	10	56.1	21.3	15.8 y
Bolognini et al. (2013)	PLP	8	59.0	1.6	>2 mo
Yoon et al. (2013)	post-SCI NP	16	44.1	2.3	>3 mo
Kumru et al. (2013)	post-SCI NP	18	49.4	8.3	>3 mo

PLP: phantom limb pain; TGNP: trigeminal neuropathic pain; CPSP: central post-stroke pain; post-SCI NP: post-spinal cord injury neuropathic pain; PNP: peripheral neuropathic pain; BPL: brachial plexus lesion; mo: months; y: years; NA: not assessed.

Although the past history of periodically cumulative rTMS sessions builds up a lasting 'memory', resulting in increased facilitation to subsequent TMS-induced neuromodulation (Valero-Cabre et al., 2008) and subsequently a prolonged analgesic effect, research in thoracic complete and incomplete SCI subjects suffering from chronic NP applying 5 daily sessions of 1Hz rTMS (1000 pulses/session) (Kang et al. 2009) or 10 daily 5Hz rTMS (500 pulses/session) (Defrin et al., 2007) showed that the intensity of pain was similarly alleviated after each treatment session of active and sham rTMS. However, the effect of time on the score for worst pain at one week after the end of the rTMS period (Kang et al., 2009) and also the pain rating index according to McGill Pain Questionnaire by the end of the 10 sessions and follow-up period of 4.5 weeks (Defrin et al., 2007) was significant with real stimulation only suggestive of a long-lasting subclinical effect.

A multicenter, randomized, double-blind, sham-controlled, crossover study in a large mixed group of patients with chronic central and peripheral NP (stroke, spinal cord injury, phantom limb, root avulsion and peripheral nerve injury) demonstrated that 10 daily 5 Hz rTMS (500 pulses/session) of M1 was tolerable and provided significant short-term pain relief although no cumulative effects have been observed (Hosomi et al., 2013b).

On the contrary, 5 daily sessions of 20Hz rTMS (2000 pulses/session) in 48 patients with unilateral chronic NP (24 had trigeminal neuralgia and 24 had post-stroke pain) (Khedr et al., 2004) and 10Hz rTMS (1000 pulses/session) over M1 in central post-stroke pain patients (Ohn et al., 2012) proved to produce long lasting pain relief for about 2 weeks when compared to sham-rTMS.

Also, by applying 5 consecutive sessions of 20Hz rTMS (1500 pulses/session) in diabetic patients with chronic drug-resistant NP using a H-coil that allows direct activation of deeper neuronal populations to induce analgesic effect is more consistent, lasting about 3 weeks (Onesti et al., 2013), suggesting that using devices allowing more focalized magnetic stimulation and also increasing the number of pulses per session can lead to more consistent pain modulation effects in selected group of patients.

Repetitive TMS over Non-Motor Cortex for Neuropathic Pain

Alterations in activity of cerebral structures involved in pain perception and pain modulation, such as the prefrontal and somatosensory cortex, have been described in patients with central (Henry et al., 2008) and peripheral NP (Cauda et al., 2009) but little work has focused on the potential role of magnetic stimulation of non-motor cerebral areas in the management of NP.

Table 2. Summary of neuropathic pain characteristics and main treatment outcomes of different protocols of rTMS

Authors (year)	Subject population	Pain intensity at baseline (NRS)	Pain measurements	Treatment protocol	Results	Adverse effects	Follow-up
Topper et al. (2003)	PLP	48.7/100	VAS	15 sessions/ 10 Hz or 1 Hz rTMS/ 110% of RMT/ 400 and 720 pulses respectively/ S1	57.7% of pain reduction with 10 Hz and 32.3% with 1 Hz after each session.	NA	NA
Khedr et al. (2004)	TGNP, CPSP	8/10	VAS, LANSS	5 sessions/ 20 Hz rTMS/ 80% of RMT/ 2000 pulses/ M1	45% of pain reduction at the end and 40% 2 weeks later.	No adverse	2 weeks
Hirayama et al. (2006)	CPSP, post-SCI NP, TGNP, PNP	8.1/10	VAS	1 session/ 5 Hz rTMS or sham/ 90% of RMT/ 500 pulses/ S1, premotor cortex or SMA	30.2% of pain reduction	No adverse	3 hours
Andre-Obadia et al. (2006)	CPSP, post-SCI NP, PNP	NA	NRS	1 session/ 20 Hz or sham rTMS/ 90% of RMT/ 1600 pulses/ M1	14.6% pain reduction for active rTMS versus 2.9% for sham rTMS.	NA	2 weeks
Lefaucheur et al. (2008)	TGNP, NP secondary to lesion of the brachial plexus, CPSP, post-SCI NP	6.5/10	VAS, Thermal thresholds	1 session/ 10 Hz vs 1 Hz or sham rTMS/ 90% of RMT/ 1200 pulses/ M1	The mean decrease of the ongoing pain induced by 10 Hz rTMS was greater in patients with TGNP (31.8%) than in patients with NP due to brachial plexus lesion	NA	NA

	Subject population	Pain intensity at baseline (NRS)	Pain measurements	Treatment protocol	Results	Adverse effects	Follow-up
					(25.7%), thalamic stroke (16.7%) or SCI (22.7%). No effect under 1 Hz rTMS or sham.		
Borckardt et al. (2009)	PNP	6.6/10	NRS, Thermal and mechanical pain threshold	3 sessions/ 10 Hz rTMS or sham/ 100% of RMT/ 4000 pulses/ left DLPFC	19% of pain reduction. Increased heat sensory threshold and decreased cold sensory threshold.	NA	2 weeks
Kang et al. (2009)	post-SCI NP	6.3/10	NRS, BPI	5 sessions/ 10 Hz rTMS or sham/ 80% of the RMT/ 1000 pulses/ M1	Only 14.1% reduction for worst pain at 1week and 20.7% at 3weeks	NA	7 weeks
Sampson et al. (2011)	post-SCI NP, PLP, PNP	7.3/10	VAS	15 sessions/ 1 Hz rTMS/ ?% of RMT/ 1600 pulses/ right DLPFC	22.2% of pain reduction after 1 week of treatment, 26% after 3weeks and 23% at 3 months of follow-up	Discomfort, headache	3 months
Matsumura et al (2012)	CPSP	6.8/10	VAS	1 session/ 5 Hz or sham rTMS/ 100% of RMT / 500 stimulations/ M1	17.4% of pain decrement under real rTMS and 3.1% under sham rTMS	NA	1 day
Lefaucheur et al. (2012)	TGNP, NP secondary to BPL, CPSP, post-SCI NP	8.0/10	VAS, SICI, ICF, MEP	1 session/ 10 Hz rTMS / 90% of AMT/ 2000 pulses/ M1 preceded or not by iTBS or cTBS/ 80% of AMT/ 600pulses/ M1	0% of pain decrement when TBS was used as a single protocol versus 41% and 31%, respectively, when iTBS and cTBS were combined with 10 Hz rTMS. At 1week: 20% of pain	No adverse	1 week

Table 2. (Continued)

	Subject population	Pain intensity at baseline (NRS)	Pain measurements	Treatment protocol	Results	Adverse effects	Follow-up
					decrement without priming and by 33% following iTBS priming and by 28% following cTBS priming. Decreased MEP amplit in cTBS-rTMS.		
Jette et al. (2013)	post-SCI NP	4.25/10	NRS	1 session/ 10 Hz or sham rTMS / 90 and 110% of RMT/ 2000 pulses/ M1	11.5% of pain reduction at 48h post-rTMS More pronounced pain reduction in incomplete SCI (21%) vs complete SCI (3%).	NA	1 week
Ohn et al. (2012)	CPSP	6.6/10	VAS	5 sessions/ 10 Hz rTMS/ 90% of RMT/ 1000 pulses/ M1	14% of pain reduction	NA	2 weeks
Onesti et al. (2013)	Diabeticneuropathy	66.2/100	VAS, RIII, LEP DN4, MPQ, NPSI	5 sessions/ 20 Hz or sham rTMS/ 80% of RMT/ 1500 pulses / M1	35% of pain reduction under active rTMS and 7.8% following sham stimulation at the end of the treatment. Also 25% of RIII area reduction following active rTMS and 4.7% in the sham group. Significant effect at 3 weeks of follow-up.	No adverse	3 weeks

	Subject population	Pain intensity at baseline (NRS)	Pain measurements	Treatment protocol	Results	Adverse effects	Follow-up
Hosomi et al. (2013)a	CPSP	7.8/10	NRS, RMT, MEP, CSP, SICI, ICF	1 session/ 5 Hz rTMS/ 90% of RMT/ 500pulses/ M1	>30% pain reduction in 38% of subjects ICF increased by 60% in responders	No adverse	NA
Hosomi et al. (2013)b	CPSP, post-SCI NP, PNP	75.6 /100	VAS, MPQ, PGICS	10 sessions/ 5 Hz rTMS or sham/ 90% of RMT/ 500 pulses/ M1	6.51% of pain reduction vs 2.44% just after stimulation, and 3.38% vs 0.66% 60 min after stimulation. The defined positive effect (>10% of pain reduction) was observed in 19.7% of patients.	Deterioration of squeezing, headache, numbness, hypoglycemia, anxiety, appetite loss, dizziness.	17 days

PLP: phantom limb pain; TGNP: trigeminal neuropathic pain; CPSP: central post-stroke pain; post-SCI NP: post-spinal cord injury pain; PNP: peripheral neuropathic pain; VAS: visual analog scale; NRS: numerical rating scale; LANS: Leeds assessment of neuropathic symptoms and signs scale; BPI: Brief pain inventory; DN4: Neuropathic pain diagnostic questionnaire; MPQ: McGill pain questionnaire; NPSI: Neuropathic pain symptom inventory; PGICS: Patients′ global impression of change; SICI: short interval intracortical inhibition; ICF: intracortical facilitation; MEP: motor evoked potential; CSP: cortical silent period; RIII: nociceptive flexion reflex; LEP: laser evoked potential; RMT: resting motor threshold; AMT: active motor threshold; M1: primary motor cortex; S1: primary somatosensory cortex; DLPFC: dorsolateral prefrontal cortex; SMA: supplementary motor cortex; NA: not assessed.

Table 3. Summary of neuropathic pain characteristics and main treatment outcomes of different protocols of tDCS

Authors (year)	Subject population	Pain intensity at baseline (NRS)	Pain measurements	Treatment protocol	Results	Adverse effects	Follow-up
Fregni et al. (2006)	post-SCI NP	6.1/10	VAS, Pain Global Assessment	5 sessions/ anodal-tDCS or sham (2 mA, 20 min)/ M1	40.6% of pain reduction after the 5th session. No effect during follow up.	Headache, itching under the electrodes.	16 days
Antal et al. (2010)	TGNP, CPSP, back pain, fibromyalgia	6.4/10	VAS, SICI, LICI, ICF, SICF	5 sessions/ anodal-tDCS or sham (1 mA, 20 min)/ M1	VAS decreased by 11-36.5% under anodal-tDCS and 1% decrease or 23% increase under sham stimulation on days 3-28. There were 63% responders (reduction of 30% or more in the VAS after 5 sessions) in the anodal-tDCS group and only 16% in the sham group.Decreased intracortical inhibition.	Tingling sensation, headache, fatigue, acute sleeping disturbances	1 months

Authors (year)	Subject population	Pain intensity at baseline (NRS)	Pain measurements	Treatment protocol	Results	Adverse effects	Follow-up
Soler et al. (2010)	post-SCI NP	7/10	VAS, NPSI, BPI	10 sessions/ anodal-tDCS or sham (2 mA, 20 min) with or without visual illusion/ M1	29.7% of pain decrement after the last session of treatment with respect to baseline in the tDCS + visual illusion group as well as 29% and 26.6% at 2 and 4 wk of follow-up	Headache, tiredness, transient increase in NP	2, 4,12 weeks
Dos Santos et al. (2012)	TGNP	4/10	VAS, thermal threshold	1 session/ anodal-tDCS or sham	No change in pain on VAS.	NA	NA
				sham (2 mA, 20 min)/ M1	36.2% of improvement on the threshold for experimental cold pain in the trigeminal allodynic area, mandibular branch.		

Table 3. (Continued)

Authors (year)	Subject population	Pain intensity at baseline (NRS)	Pain measurements	Treatment protocol	Results	Adverse effects	Follow-up
Wrigley et al. (2012)	post-SCI NP	5.6/10	VAS	5 sessions/ /anodal-tDCS or sham (2 mA, 20 min)/ M1	No effect	Local redness, tingling sensations, fatigue, lightheadedness, headache, sleepiness, Rarely: alertness-concentration, tension-anxiety, depression-dejection, vigour-activity, anger-hostility, confusion-bewilderment, and insomnia	1 and 6 months
Bolognini et al. (2013)	PLP	26/100	VAS	1 session/ anodal, cathodal-tDCS or sham (2 mA, 15 min)/ M1 or PPC.	M1 56% of pain decrement following anodal-tDCS over M1	No adverse	1.5 hours
Yoon et al. (2013)	post-SCI NP	7.4/10	VAS, PGICS, PET	20 session/ anodal-tDCS or sham (2 mA, 20 min) twice a day/ M1	22.9% of pain decrement after active tDCS. Increased metabolism in the medulla and decreased metabolism in the left DLPFC. No change on PGICS	NA	NA

Authors (year)	Subject population	Pain intensity at baseline (NRS)	Pain measurements	Treatment protocol	Results	Adverse effects	Follow-up
Kumru et al. (2013)	post-SCI NP	7.8/10	NRS, CHEP, Evoked heat pain, QTT	10 sessions/ anodal-tDCS (2 mA, 20 min) with visual illusion therapy/ M1	37.4% of pain reduction after anodal-tDCS and also a decrement in N2/P2 amplitude of CHEPs and subjective evoked pain vs baseline	NA	NA

PLP: phantom limb pain; TGNP: trigeminal neuropathic pain; CPSP: central post-stroke pain; post-SCI NP: post-spinal cord injury pain; VAS: visual analog scale; NRS: numerical rating scale; BPI: Brief pain inventory; NPSI: Neuropathic pain symptom inventory; PGICS: Patients' global impression of change; SICI: short interval intracortical inhibition; LICI: long interval intracortical inhibition; ICF: intracortical facilitation; SICF: short interval intracortical facilitation; PET: positron emission tomography; CHEP: contact heat evoked potential; M1: primary motor cortex; PPC: primary parietal cortex; NA: not assessed. mA: miliamper; M1: motor cortex.

Sampson et al. (2011) reported a greater than 50% decline in pain ratings by the completion of 15 sessions of 1Hz rTMS (1600 stimulations/session) applied to the right DLPFC rTMS as an adjuvant treatment in 3 out of 9 subjects with refractory NP in (Sampson et al., 2011). Similarly to the effects of rTMS over M1, magnetic stimulation of DLPFC at higher frequencies and also increasing the number of magnetic pulses per session was associated with more consistent pain modulation as confirmed by a consistent 19% decrease in daily average pain lasting about 2 weeks in four participants with chronic peripheral NP following a series of 3 sessions of 10 Hz rTMS (4000 pulses/session) of left DLPFC (Borckardt et al., 2011).

In spite of the fact that M1 and S1 are located adjacently and recent research showed that modulation of M1 can induce detectable electrophysiologic changes in S1 following TBS (Murakami et al., 2008) and low frequency rTMS in healthy subjects (Kodama et al., 2009), only two studies has been carried out in patients with NP to target the S1 for rTMS. However, both studies failed to induce analgesia in patients with peripheral NP following a single session of 5 Hz rTMS (Hirayama et al., 2006) or 15 session of 1Hz or 10Hz rTMS of the S1 (Topper et al., 2003).

Mechanisms of rTMS-Induced Modulation in Neuropathic Pain

Neuropathic pain state can develop following complex maladaptive neuroplastic changes affecting nociception and pain modulation. Whereas post-stroke pain is associated with injury to the spinothalamic tract, thalamus, or thalamocortical tract which determine alteration of afferent input and dysregulation of cortical excitability (Dostrovsky, 2000; Frese et al., 2006). NP secondary to SCI is related to metabolic alterations of the Glutamate/Myo-inositol ratio in the anterior cingulate and prefrontal cortex (Stanwell et al., 2010; Widerstrom-Noga et al., 2013), as well as functional hyperactivity of the anterior cingulate, insula, DLPFC, premotor cortex and supplementary motor area (Gustin, 2010). These alterations are considered to contribute essentially to the mechanism of central sensitization of NP. Furthermore, the decrease in intracortical inhibition in central post stroke pain (Hosomi et al., 2013a) as well as in post-SCI pain subjects (Lefaucheur et al., 2006) and its restoration following high-frequency rTMS points to the GABA-ergic neurotransmission recovery as a potential neurobiological mechanism of this technique underlying pain relief. However, the analgesic effect of rTMS seems not to be associated exclusively with excitability alterations at the motor cortex level itself since no specific differences in the motor evoked potential amplitude was observed following high-frequency magnetic stimulation of the M1 corresponding to painful or non-painful area (Jette et al., 2013) or by the motor evoked potential recruitment curve under low-frequency rTMS (Wassermann et al., 1998). Also, no correlation has been observed between the current perception and the excitability in S1 under low-frequency rTMS as measured by somatosensory evoked potentials (Kodama et al., 2009).

Functional MRI data demonstrated that 10 Hz rTMS applied over the right M1 in healthy subjects elicited significant deactivation in many cerebral structure including: the right superior and middle frontal gyri, bilateral postcentral and bilateral cingulate gyri, left supplementary motor area, right insula, right basal ganglia, and right cerebellar hemisphere but only the deactivation of the sensory network was associated with an increase in the sensory threshold (Yoo et al., 2008). When applying the same frequency in post-stroke pain patients a significant decreased activity was observed in the secondary somatosensory cortex, insula, prefrontal cortex, and putamen on fMRI. However, the antalgic effect was more prominent in patients with more preserved superior talamocortical tract in the ipsilesional hemisphere which showed significant correlation with change of pain score after 5 daily sessions of 10Hz rTMS supporting the role of the intact pathways in modulating analgesia mechanism (Ohn et al., 2012).

High frequency rTMS of the M1 also determines distant effects such as top-down activation of brainstem periaqueductal gray matter and rostral ventromedial medulla driving descending inhibition. This hypothesis is supported by observations that deep 20Hz rTMS of M1 cortex can markedly inhibit spinal cord reflexes in patients with peripheral NP (Onesti et al., 2013) or with incomplete spinal cord injury (Jette et al., 2013) and the analgesic effect can be decreased following Naloxone administration (de Andrade et al., 2010). However, studies in healthy volunteers failed to show effect on the threshold or recruitment curve of the nociceptive flexion reflex following 10 Hz rTMS of M1 (Nahmias et al., 2009) although contribution of factors such as the differences in applied frequencies and metaplasticity phenomena to differential neuromodulation effects in NP patients and healthy subjects cannot be excluded. Indeed, neurons have a striking tendency to engage in oscillatory activities. Oscillatory activity in the beta-frequency band (13-35 Hz) can be recorded over the sensory and motor cortex in human and functional coupling of sensory and motor cortices in the beta-band was confirmed in electrocorticographic recordings of in patients with chronic pain syndromes, suggesting a means by which beta-activity may simultaneously influence cortical sensory-motor interaction (Baker, 2007; Lalo et al., 2007; Pogosyan et al., 2009). Frequency-related distant effects of rTMS are also supported by animal studies showing that only multiple sessions of high-frequency rTMS induces neuroplastic changes as measured by BDNF and GluR1 in the brain, whereas low-frequency rTMS has no long-term effects on these markers (Gersner et al., 2011). Moreover, 25 Hz but not sham rTMS for 8 weeks in SCI rats reduced about 30% the Iba1 and GFAP, markers of spinal dorsal horn microglia and astrocytes activation reported to contribute to hyper-responsive states in cases of chronic NP (Kim et al., 2013).

rTMS over the DLPFC share some similar mechanisms with the magnetic stimulation of M1 although it seems to determine side-related differences of neuromodulation. The application of 10Hz rTMS over the left DLPFC in healthy subjects was associated with increased activity in several areas, including the right superior frontal gyrus and insula, anterior and posterior cingulate gyri and brainstem. Increased superior frontal activity was significantly associated with decreased pain intensity ratings (Martin et al., 2013) and can be blocked by Naloxone pretreatment suggesting that endogenous opioidergic system mediated this effect (Taylor et al., 2012). On the contrary, unilateral 10Hz rTMS of the right DLPFC induces diffuse and selective analgesic effects over the experimental pain in healthy volunteers but lacks of modulation effects on the RIII reflex (Nahmias et al., 2009). Also, Naloxone injection had no effects on rTMS-induced analgesia following the right DLPFC rTMS in another study (de Andrade et al., 2010) suggesting that modulation effects of the right and left DLPFC magnetic stimulation are mediated by different mechanisms. Unlike Naloxone, which blocks only the analgesic effects elicited by M1 stimulation, ketamine decreased the effects of both 10Hz rTMS of the right M1 and DLPFC stimulation in healthy subjects without alterations of cortical excitability parameters (resting motor threshold, suprathreshold motor evoked potentials, short intracortical inhibition, and intracortical facilitation), suggesting that a final common pathway may underlie the analgesia induced by the stimulation of these two cortical sites. Furthermore, these results are consistent with a role for long-term potentiation-like phenomena in this type of analgesia (Ciampi de Andrade et al., 2014).

In spite of the fact that M1 and S1 are located adjacently and modulation of M1 can induce high-frequency oscillations changes in S1 following intermittent TBS and continuous TBS (Murakami et al., 2008) as well as decreased amplitudes of P25/N33 component of the somatosensory evoked potentials following low-frequency rTMS of M1 (Kodama et al., 2009), direct S1 modulation by either intermittent TBS, intermediate TBS or continuous TBS showed no pain modulation effects in healthy subjects (Poreisz et al., 2008). However, a mechanistic relation between S1 plasticity and pain-relieving effects is far from being established although the decreased amplitudes of P25/N33 component of the somatosensory evoked potentials following continues TBS over S1 (Ishikawa et al., 2007) as well as the diminished amplitude of the N2 component oflaser evoked potentials following either intermittent TBS, intermediate TBS or continuous TBS (Poreisz et al., 2008) indicate that subclinical modulation effects over the nociceptive and non-nociceptive pathway function have been induced by these techniques.

Combination of rTMS with Other Treatments

The analgesic effects of 'conventional' 10Hz-rTMS delivered to M1 can be enhanced by TBS priming. Using iTBS priming tends to enhance the analgesic effects that are produced in patients with chronic NP by 10Hz-rTMS delivered to M1, whereas TBS applied as a single protocol cannot relieve pain (Lefaucheur et al., 2012). However, it is not clear whether the TBS priming generates a simple additive effect or a more specific process of cortical plasticity.

The relationship between pharmacologic background and the effects of 5Hz rTMS of the M1 revealed that rTMS-induced analgesia correlated well with pain reduction by ketamine, morphine, and thiopental in central post-stroke pain patients. However, ketamine sensitivity was observed in more cases compared with morphine and thiopental. Therefore, such a combination treatment determined on the basis of the drug challenge test may be useful for enhancing rTMS-induced analgesia in poststroke pain patients (Matsumura et al., 2013).

Safety and Side Effects of TMS

Although the TMS is generally considered secure there are safety considerations, particularly when TMS pulses are applied repeatedly. The only absolute contraindication to TMS/rTMS is the presence of metallic hardware in close contact to the discharging coil (such as cochlear implants, or an Internal Pulse Generator or medication pumps). In such instances there is a risk of inducing malfunctioning of the implanted devices. However, other conditions of increased or uncertain risk of inducing epileptic seizure should also be considered (Rossi et al., 2009).

The most common adverse effect of TMS is the headache, which is reported by about 10% of subjects (Hosomi et al., 2013b; Sampson et al., 2011; Treister et al., 2013). This is attributed to the TMS coil being pressed against subjects' heads for an extended time. The TMS-induced headaches are usually mild and respond to usual headache treatments such as acetaminophen. Lastly, depending on where TMS is applied, and its intensity, suprathreshold application to the M1 can activate the facial, trigeminal, or auditory nerves to cause discomfort (Treister et al., 2013). Other adverse effects such as hypoglycemia, anxiety, appetite loss, dizziness have rarely been described (Hosomi et al., 2013b).

Transcranial Direct Current Stimulation (tDCS)

tDCS is a non-invasive technique of neuromodulation based on the application of a weak direct current (1-2 mA) to the scalp that flows between two pad electrodes (anode and cathode) (DosSantos et al., 2012). The term ‘direct’ means the electrical flow is unidirectional traveling from one positive electrode (anode) towards the other negative electrode (cathode). Therefore, according to the type of electrode applied over the target cortical area tDCS is classified as anodal (anodal-tDCS) or cathodal (cathodal-tDCS) (Vaseghi et al., 2014). High-definition tDCS (HD-tDCS) is a newly developed intervention that increases the accuracy of current delivery to the brain by using arrays of smaller electrodes, instead of the larger pad electrodes of conventional tDCS. Targeting is achieved by energizing electrodes placed in predetermined configurations with a center ring electrode (anode or cathode) overlying the target cortical region and other surrounding return electrodes which help circumscribe the area of stimulation (Villamar et al., 2013).

Since pain is a multidimensional experience with sensory-discriminative, cognitive-evaluative and affective-motivational components the S1, M1 and DLPFC complexly contribute to nociception and pain modulation and therefore their stimulation using tDCS protocols could lead to a differential effect on pain symptoms relief.

tDCS over Motor Cortex for Neuropathic Pain

Similarly to the rTMS the application of a single session of tDCS proved to have short lasting neuromodolatory effects. The application of one session of anodal-tDCS of M1 failed to reduce the intensity of trigeminal NP in a case study (DosSantos et al., 2012). However, it induced 36.2% of improvement in the threshold of experimental cold pain in the trigeminal allodynic area and mandibular branch and was associated with a decreased non-displaceable biding potential of μ-opioid receptors quantified with a selective radiotracer, [11C]carfentanil suggesting that the effects of a single tDCS session are subclinical at immediate level, and repetitive sessions might be necessary to revert ingrained neuroplastic changes related to the chronic pain (DosSantos et al., 2012). Moreover, the effects of the tDCS over the M1 can be highly specific to different sensory pathways as revealed by a double-blind, sham-controlled research showing a short lasting decrease of the phantom limb pain intensity (56%), but not of the non-painful phantom limb sensations (stump pain and telescoping) followinga single session of anodal-tDCS over M1 (Bolognini et al., 2013).

Increasing the number of treatment sessions can lead to long-lasting clinical improvement. The application of 5 sessions of anodal-tDCS over M1 in consecutive days proved to be effective in lessening pain at the end of treatment and also led to a long-lasting pain relief up 4-week in duration in patients with multiple sclerosis (Mori et al., 2009), peripheral diabetic NP (Kim et al., 2014), and other therapy-resistant chronic pain syndromes (trigeminal neuralgia, post-stroke pain, back pain, fibromyalgia) (Antal et al., 2010).

However, when multiple sessions of tDCS are applied the therapeutic effects may also depend on the type and evolution of the NP being treated. When anodal-tDCS (2mA, 20 min) of M1 was applied for 5 consecutive days in 8 subjects with complete and 3 subjects with incomplete traumatic SCI (3.5 years of evolution) presenting central NP for more than 3 months, a significant pain improvement was observed after active but not sham stimulation. In the follow-up (16 days), however, there was only a trend toward a significant difference between baseline versus follow-up (Fregni et al., 2006). On the contrary, a similar treatment protocol did not provide any short-term or long-term pain relief in a group of patients with complete SCI with longer evolution of the chronic central NP (15.8 years) (Wrigley et al., 2013).

Increasing the number of anodal-tDCS sessions to 10 daily sessions during two consecutive weeks and combining it with virtual reality in SCI patients (80% with complete and 20% with incomplete SCI) with non-homogenous evolution of the spinal lesion (1 to 31 years) and refractory NP, Soler et al. (2010) observed a significant relief of the continuous and paroxismal pain on the last day of treatment in the active group, and the effect was long-lasting (up to 4 weeks) for the paroxysmal pain only. Interestingly, when the anodal-tDCS over M1 was combined with walking visual illusion patients experienced a significant improvement in all pain subtypes (continuous and paroxysmal pain, allodynia and dysesthesia) at the end of treatment as well as during follow-up. At 12 weeks after treatment, the combined treatment group still presented significant improvement on the overall pain intensity perception; whereas no improvements were reported in the other groups (Soler et al., 2010). Furthermore, two weeks of non-invasive stimulation also induced significant decrease of pain intensity (>50%) in 72% of SCI patients with NP undergoing tDCS associated with virtual illusion and also determined significant changes in contact heat evoked potentials amplitude, evoked pain and heat pain threshold with respect to baseline (Kumru et al., 2012). However, the higer degree of pain relief in the study of Kumru et al. (2012) compared to the study published by Soler et al. (2010) might be related to differences in clinical characteristics of the population undegoing tDCS since in the study of Kumru et al. (2012) 83% of the patients presented incomplete SCI, and the NP was mainly subacute in evolution and the tDCS was first choice for NP before any other medication in few patients.

Interestingly, when a double number of anodal-tDCS (2 mA, 20 min) sessions was applied during the same time period (10 days) in patients with non-refractory NP (>3 months of evolution) secondary to traumatic complete and incomplete SCI of relatively recent evolution (2.3 years), subjects in the active treatment group rated their intensity of pain as reduced by 22.9% at the end of treatment with respect to baseline and pain interference with general daily life was smaller than in the sham treated group. However, pain reduction was higher in incomplete (35%) than complete SCI subjects (13%) (Yoon et al., 2013). Differences in treatment outcomes following tDCS are also supported by results of a recent Cochrane review including 5 studies (83 subjects) suggesting that therapeutic effects of the anodal tDCS over M1 in chronic pain is observed only when studying homogenous groups (O'Connell et al., 2011).

tDCS over Non-Motor Brain Areas for Neuropathic Pain

Five daily sessions of anodal-tDCS over the DLPFC (20 min, 2 mA) can alleviate peripheral diabetic NP at short (immediately after) and long-term (two weeks after the treatment). However, the long-lasting analgesic effect is shorter than in protocols targeting the M1 cortex and no changes in Clinical Global Impression score, anxiety, depression, sleep quality, and the pain to pressure threshold are associated (Kim et al., 2014).

The effectiveness of cathodal over anodal tDCS to modulate sensory functioning when applied over the S1 has been confirmed recently in subjects with NP. Cathodal but not anodal tDCS (2 mA, 15 min)or sham stimulation of S1 determined a short-lasting decrease of non-painful phantom limb sensations (Bolognini et al., 2013) wherease application of either cathodal-tDCS over the S1 or anodal-tDCS over the M1 (2mA, 20 min, every other day during 5 consecutive days) resulted in a moderate reduction of the itching sensation in a patient with syringomyelia (Knotkova et al., 2013). Both studies suggest possible polarity-specific modulation of somatosensory cortical plasticity related with non-painful sensations with no effects on NP. However, a more extended meta-analysis including 13 studies on patients with different forms of chronic pain revealed that anodal-tDCS of M1 or DLPFC but not of S1 produced significant pain modulation when compared with sham stimulation (Vaseghi et al., 2014). The average decrease in visual analogue score was 14.9% and 19.3% after applying anodal-tDCS on the M1 and DLPFC respectively although compared to stimulation of M1, the effect size after applying anodal-tDCS on DLPFC is bigger (Vaseghi et al., 2014).

Combination of tDCS with Other Treatments

Based on observations that both movement imagery and movement itself activate similar brain regions (Pascual-Leone et al., 2005) and also cause an increase in corticospinal excitability and a decrease in intracortical inhibition (Kumru et al., 2008). The combination of anodal-tDCS over M1 with techniques of visual illusion proved to have a synergic effect. Indeed, SCI patients receiving anodal-tDCS and visual illusion experienced a significant improvement in continuous and paroxismal pain as well as in allodynia and dysesthesia which were more prominent and also longer-lasting in comparison to any of those interventions alone or to placebo (Soler et al., 2010). Also, preconditioning the 1Hz rTMS applied over M1 with weak tDCS (1 mA) in healthy subjects showed that cathodal preconditioning successfully reversed the normal suppressive effect of low-frequency rTMS and effectively modulated cold and heat pain thresholds (Moloney and Witney, 2012). Conversely, anodal preconditioning of the rTMS led to a decrease in cold pain thresholds suggesting that preconditioning M1 using cathodal-tDCS before subsequent stimulation via 1Hz rTMS facilitates the production of analgesia (Moloney and Witney, 2012). On the other hand, concurrent application of neuromuscular electrical stimulation (NMES) and cathodal-tDCS (protocols that reduces cortical excitability when applied alone) suppressed the enhanced cortical excitation induced by NMES alone suggesting that careful testing of combined interventions is necessary before application in clinical contexts (Schabrun et al., 2012). tDCS may also improve pain control through neuromodulation of the endogenous pain modulation systems (Reidler et al., 2012). Anodal-tDCS and the descending noxious inhibitory controls paradigm significantly increased pain thresholds in healthy subjects suggesting that existing pain therapies involving DNIC may be enhanced through combination with non-invasive brain stimulation (Reidler et al., 2012).

Mechanisms of tDCS-Induced Modulation in Neuropathic Pain

The mechanisms underlying effects of tDCS are believed to be complex involving changes in spontaneous neuronal firing rates, synaptic and non-synaptic plasticity and changes of resting polarization of the neurons. These effects depend upon factors such as: the size, polarity and position of the electrodes, the applied current intensity, the density and duration of stimulation, and the properties of the tissue in the stimulated area (Medeiros et al., 2013).

It is generally assumed that anodal-tDCS has an excitatory effect on limited cortical areas by depolarizing neurons, while the converse applies to the cathode through the process of hyperpolarization (Gomez Palacio Schjetnan et al., 2013). Prolonged or strong stimulation, however, may determine opposite effects, resulting in diminished excitability after the anodal-tDCS and enhanced excitability after the cathodal-tDCS (Batsikadze et al., 2013; Monte-Silva et al., 2010). Furthermore, whereas the position of the electrodes appears to be critical for determining the direction and spatial distribution of the current flow, the direction of polarization seems to depend strictly on the orientation of axons and dendrites in the induced electrical field (Zaghi et al., 2009).

Most of the studies indicate that the polarity-driven alterations of resting membrane potentials represent the crucial mechanisms of the tDCS-induced effects (Liebetanz et al., 2002; Nitsche et al., 2002). Indeed, magnetic resonance spectroscopy provided evidence that excitatory anodal-tDCS causes locally reduction of GABA while inhibitory cathodal-tDCS causes reduced glutamatergic neuronal activity (Stagg et al., 2014). However, beyond regional effects under the electrodes, there are activity alterations of interconnected remote cortical and subcortical areas involving modulation of the opioid (DosSantos et al., 2012), dopamine (Kuo et al., 2008; Monte-Silva et al., 2009), acetylcholine (Kuo et al., 2007) and serotonin (Nitsche et al., 2009). Furthermore, single or multiple tDCS sessions seems to involve differential mechanims of neuroplasticity. Single anodal-tDCS application over the M1 in a trigeminal neuropathic pain patient immediately increases functional coupling between ipsilateral M1 and thalamus whereas cathodal-tDCS decreases functional coupling between ipsilateral M1 and contralateral putamen (DosSantos et al., 2012). The considerably decreased non-displaceable binding potential of the carfentanil (a μ1-opioid receptor selective radiotracer) in subcortical pain-matrix structures compared to sham-tDCS, especially in the posterior thalamus, suggest that the analgesic effect of M1-tDCS is possibly due to direct polarity-dependent increase of endogenous opioid release (DosSantos et al., 2012). However, widespread modulation in cortical and subcortical areas, including in the underlying M1, contralateral frontal and primary sensorimotor cortex have also been observed irrespective of polarity (Lang et al., 2005).

The tDCS polarity-dependent effects elicited during the application of the anodal-tDCS are far less prominent than the after-effects of anodal-tDCS, whereas the effects evoked during and after cathodal-tDCS are very similar. Specifically, for the short-lasting after-effects (7 min tDCS), inhibition is diminished and facilitation increased by anodal-tDCS suggesting that the after-effects of tDCS are at least partly controlled by NMDA receptor activity (Nitsche et al., 2005). However, the after-effects of tDCS have also a non-synaptic mechanism of action based upon changes in neural membrane function. These changes, apart from reflecting local changes in ionic concentrations, could arise from alterations in transmembrane proteins and from electrolysis-related changes in [H+] induced by exposure to constant electric field (Ardolino et al., 2005).

Functional coupling between the M1 and subcortical structures involved in pain perception and pain modulation is supposed to be another important mechanism that determines the tDCS-related analgesia. The activation of thalamic nuclei directly connected with motor and premotor cortices entail a cascade of synaptic events in pain-related structures receiving afferents from the medial thalamus, anterior cingulate and upper brainstem (Garcia-Larrea et al., 1999). At the same time the motor cortex stimulation using direct currents can modulate emotional and cognitive components of pain and normalize excessive attention to pain and pain-related information through functional modulation of the anterior cingulate cortex and insula (Yoon et al., 2013). Indeed, anodal-tDCS in healthy subjects determined an increase in pain threshold after anodal-tDCS which was negatively correlated with baseline glutamine levels in the thalamus and positively correlated with baseline N-acetylaspartate in the cingulate cortex as measured by magnetic resonance spectroscopy (Reidler et al., 2012).

Given that the DLPFC is involved in the affective dimension of pain experience, its activation through non-invasive techniques could modulate affective-emotional networks regulating the unpleasantness associated with pain symptoms as well as may trigger descending pain inhibitory mechanisms via an indirect, inhibitory effect on the thalamus. Human study using anodal-tDCS over the left DLPFC revealed an increased activation of regions closely anatomically connected to the DLPFC in conjunction with a decreased functional coupling between the homolateral DLPFC and the thalami bilaterally (Stagg et al., 2013) which are associated with decrease in subjective reports of emotional and sensory aspects of pain (Maeoka et al., 2012). Therefore, stimulation of DLPFC could modulate the affective component of chronic pain, attenuating unpleasantness and emotional discomfort while related to historical personal experience via its cognitive-evaluative role (Plow et al., 2012).

Safety and Side Effects of tDCS

Overall, tDCS is considered a safe and painless technique for electrically stimulating the brain. MRI performed in healthy subjects at 30 and 60 min after tDCS did not show pathological signal alterations such us brain edema or alterations of the blood-brain barrier or cerebral tissue damage detectable in post-contrast-enhanced T1-weighted and diffusion-weighted MRI sequences (Nitsche et al., 2004). However, a comprehensive research (Poreisz et al., 2007) summarizing the partially adverse effects of 567 tDCS sessions over motor and non-motor cortical areas from different research including healthy subjects (75% of studies) and patients (25% of studies) with migraine , stroke and tinnitus revealed that during tDCS a mild tingling sensation was the most common reported adverse effect (70.6%), followed by moderate fatigue that was felt by 35.3% of the subjects, and a light itching sensation under the stimulation electrodes reported by 30.4% of the subjects. Headache (11.8%), nausea (2.9%) and insomnia (0.98%) were also reported after tDCS, but fairly infrequently. Interestingly, the incidence of the itching sensation and the intensity of tingling sensation were significantly higher during tDCS in the group of the healthy subjects, in comparison to patients; whereas the occurrence of headache was significantly higher in the patients group after the stimulation (Poreisz et al., 2007). Moreover, the electrochemical products generated by the currents contact the skin and tissue heating may result in skin irritation and skin burning (Palm et al., 2008).

Discussion

Non-invasive brain stimulation techniques such as tDCS and rTMS proved to be useful tools to modulate brain activity and to correct the maladaptive neuroplastic changes related to chronic pain disorders. There is strong evidence that application of series of rTMS sessions on consecutive days as well as stimulation at high-frequencies is associated with more prominent analgesic effect assumed to lead to the build-up of cumulative effects (Borckardt et al., 2011). However, in addition to the key parameters that define rTMS trains (intensity, frequency, train duration, and inter-train interval), the repeated application of rTMS introduces supplementary dosing parameters that describe the cumulative exposure to rTMS. These include total pulses per session, sessions per day, days per week, weeks per acute course, and maintenance frequency (Rossi et al., 2009). Therefore, the high variability of these factors may determine a different course for neuroplastic phenomena following the application of multiple sessions of rTMS. In addition, the existing research also suggest that rTMS may have a differential analgesic effect based on neuroanatomical origins of the NP pathophysiology and the integrity of the neuromodulatory pathways with more effective treatment response observed in NP states originating from the ''top'' (supraspinal, cranial or spinal) than the ''bottom'' (nerve root or peripheral nerve) locations in the overall cranio-caudal neuroanatomical scheme as the greates treatment was calculated for trigeminal neuropathic pain, followed by post-stroke supraspinal related pain, spinal cord injury related pain, nerve root and peripheral nerve pain according to a recent meta-analysis (Leung et al., 2009).

Regarding the use of tDCS as a treatment for chronic pain research indicate that anodal-tDCS over the M1 can be effective for specific forms of pain, particularly for NP related to incomplete spinal cord injury patients with a recent evolution. The analgesic effects induced by tDCS has been shown to outlast the period of stimulation and are cumulative therefore options to prolong the effects of tDCS are further prolongation or repetition of tDCS sessions. Exploration ofthe effects of different break durations (0, 3, 20, 180 min or 24 hours) on cathodal-tDCS (1 mA, 9 min) induced cortical excitability alterations revealed that doubling stimulation duration without a break prolongs the after-effects from 60 to 90 min after tDCS. When the second stimulation was performed during the after-effects of the first, a prolongation and enhancement of tDCS-induced effects for ≦120 min after stimulation was observed (Monte-Silva et al., 2010). In contrast, when the second stimulation followed the first one after 3 or 24 h, the aftere-ffects were initially attenuated, or abolished, but afterwards reestablished for up to 120 min after tDCS in the 24-h condition suggesting that specific temporal design might be important, for prolonging the after-effects of tDCS (Monte-Silva et al., 2010). Also, since the effects of tDCS appear to depend on the level of cortical excitability at the time of the stimulation, additional synergic therapeutic effect can be reached through combination of the tDCS with other therapies such as visual illusion and rTMS.

The selection of the motor cortex is the most widely used cortical target for rTMS and tDCS in the management of NP but confounding factors such as the small number of studies that used prefrontal or somatosensory cortical stimulation for pain modulation should be considered. However, tDCS of the S1 might be applied as therapy intervention for modulation of non-painful sensory symptoms associated with neuropathic pain states.

Conclusion

Despite many limitations, results of the existing researchs support the use of tDCS and rTMS as non-invasive stimulation techniques for the treatment of neuropathic pain syndromes in selected patient populations. Both rTMS and tDCS are easy to apply and have been shown to be safe, with few and usually mild adverse effect.

References

Abraham, WC; Tate, WP. Metaplasticity: a new vista across the field of synaptic plasticity. *Prog Neurobiol*, 1997, 52, 303-323.

Andre-Obadia, N; Peyron, R; Mertens, P; Mauguiere, F; Laurent, B; Garcia-Larrea, L. Transcranial magnetic stimulation for pain control. Double-blind study of different frequencies against placebo, and correlation with motor cortex stimulation efficacy. *Clin Neurophysiol*, 2006, 117, 1536-1544.

Antal, A; Terney, D; Kuhnl, S; Paulus, W. Anodal transcranial direct current stimulation of the motor cortex ameliorates chronic pain and reduces short intracortical inhibition. *J Pain Symptom Manage*, 2010, 39, 890-903.

Ardolino, G; Bossi, B; Barbieri, S; Priori, A. Non-synaptic mechanisms underlie the after-effects of cathodal transcutaneous direct current stimulation of the human brain. *J Physiol*, 2005, 568, 653-663.

Baker, SN. Oscillatory interactions between sensorimotor cortex and the periphery. *Curr Opin Neurobiol*, 2007, 17, 649-655.

Baron, R. Neuropathic pain: a clinical perspective. *Handb Exp Pharmacol*, 2009, 3-30.

Batsikadze, G; Moliadze, V; Paulus, W; Kuo, MF; Nitsche, MA. Partially non-linear stimulation intensity-dependent effects of direct current stimulation on motor cortex excitability in humans. *J Physiol*, 2013, 591, 1987-2000.

Bolognini, N; Olgiati, E; Maravita, A; Ferraro, F; Fregni, F. Motor and parietal cortex stimulation for phantom limb pain and sensations. *Pain*, 2013, 154, 1274-1280.

Borckardt, JJ; Reeves, ST; Beam, W; Jensen, MP; Gracely, RH; Katz, S; et al. A randomized, controlled investigation of motor cortex transcranial magnetic stimulation (TMS) effects on quantitative sensory measures in healthy adults: evaluation of TMS device parameters. *Clin J Pain*, 2011, 27, 486-494.

Calmels, P; Mick, G; Perrouin-Verbe, B; Ventura, M. Neuropathic pain in spinal cord injury: identification, classification, evaluation. *Ann Phys Rehabil Med*, 2009, 52, 83-102.

Cauda, F; Sacco, K; Duca, S; Cocito, D; D'Agata, F; Geminiani, GC; et al. Altered resting state in diabetic neuropathic pain. PLoS One, 2009, 4, e4542.

Ciampi de Andrade, D; Mhalla, A; Adam, F; Texeira, MJ; Bouhassira, D. Repetitive transcranial magnetic stimulation induced analgesia depends on N-methyl-D-aspartate glutamate receptors. *Pain*, 2014, 155, 598-605.

Cramer, SC; Sur, M; Dobkin, BH; O'Brien, C; Sanger, TD; Trojanowski, JQ; et al. Harnessing neuroplasticity for clinical applications. *Brain*, 2011, 134, 1591-1609.

de Andrade, DC; Mhalla, A; Adam, F; Texeira, MJ; Bouhassira, D. Neuropharmacological basis of rTMS-induced analgesia: the role of endogenous opioids. *Pain*, 2010, 152, 320-326.

deCharms, RC; Maeda, F; Glover, GH; Ludlow, D; Pauly, JM; Soneji, D; et al. Control over brain activation and pain learned by using real-time functional MRI. *Proc Natl Acad Sci U S A*, 2005, 102, 18626-18631.

Defrin, R; Grunhaus, L; Zamir, D; Zeilig, G. The effect of a series of repetitive transcranial magnetic stimulations of the motor cortex on central pain after spinal cord injury. *Arch Phys Med Rehabil*, 2007, 88, 1574-1580.

Di Lazzaro, V; Dileone, M; Pilato, F; Capone, F; Musumeci, G; Ranieri, F; et al. Modulation of motor cortex neuronal networks by rTMS: comparison of local and remote effects of six different protocols of stimulation. *J Neurophysiol*, 2011, 105, 2150-2156.

DosSantos, MF; Love, TM; Martikainen, IK; Nascimento, TD; Fregni, F; Cummiford, C; et al. Immediate effects of tDCS on the mu-opioid system of a chronic pain patient. *Front Psychiatry*, 2012, 3, 93.

Dostrovsky, JO. Role of thalamus in pain. *Prog Brain Res*, 2000, 129, 245-257.

Ferguson, AR; Huie, JR; Crown, ED; Baumbauer, KM; Hook, MA; Garraway, SM; et al. Maladaptive spinal plasticity opposes spinal learning and recovery in spinal cord injury. *Front Physiol*, 2012, 3, 399.

Fregni, F; Boggio, PS; Lima, MC; Ferreira, MJ; Wagner, T; Rigonatti, SP; et al. A sham-controlled, phase II trial of transcranial direct current stimulation for the treatment of central pain in traumatic spinal cord injury. *Pain*, 2006, 122, 197-209.

Frese, A; Husstedt, IW; Ringelstein, EB; Evers, S. Pharmacologic treatment of central post-stroke pain. *Clin J Pain*, 2006, 22, 252-260.

Garcia-Larrea, L; Peyron, R; Mertens, P; Gregoire, MC; Lavenne, F; Le Bars, D; et al. Electrical stimulation of motor cortex for pain control: a combined PET-scan and electrophysiological study. *Pain*, 1999, 83, 259-273.

Gersner, R; Kravetz, E; Feil, J; Pell, G; Zangen, A. Long-term effects of repetitive transcranial magnetic stimulation on markers for neuroplasticity: differential outcomes in anesthetized and awake animals. *J Neurosci*, 2011, 31, 7521-7526.

Gomez Palacio Schjetnan, A; Faraji, J; Metz, GA; Tatsuno, M; Luczak, A. Transcranial direct current stimulation in stroke rehabilitation: a review of recent advancements. *Stroke Res Treat*, 2013, 2013, 170256.

Gustin, SM; Wrigley, PJ; Siddall, PJ; Henderson, LA. Brain anatomy changes associated with persistent neuropathic pain following spinal cord injury. *Cereb Cortex*, 2010, 20, 1409-1419.

Haanpaa, M; Attal, N; Backonja, M; Baron, R; Bennett, M; Bouhassira, D; et al. NeuPSIG guidelines on neuropathic pain assessment. *Pain*, 2011, 152, 14-27.

Henry, JL; Lalloo, C; Yashpal, K. Central poststroke pain: an abstruse outcome. *Pain Res Manag*, 2008, 13, 41-49.

Hirayama, A; Saitoh, Y; Kishima, H; Shimokawa, T; Oshino, S; Hirata, M; et al. Reduction of intractable deafferentation pain by navigation-guided repetitive transcranial magnetic stimulation of the primary motor cortex. *Pain*, 2006, 122, 22-27.

Hosomi, K; Kishima, H; Oshino, S; Hirata, M; Tani, N; Maruo, T; et al. Cortical excitability changes after high-frequency repetitive transcranial magnetic stimulation for central poststroke pain. *Pain*, 2013a, 154, 1352-1357.

Hosomi, K; Shimokawa, T; Ikoma, K; Nakamura, Y; Sugiyama, K; Ugawa, Y; et al. Daily repetitive transcranial magnetic stimulation of primary motor cortex for neuropathic pain: a randomized, multicenter, double-blind, crossover, sham-controlled trial. *Pain*, 2013b, 154, 1065-1072.

Huang, YZ; Edwards, MJ; Rounis, E; Bhatia, KP; Rothwell, JC. Theta burst stimulation of the human motor cortex. *Neuron*, 2005, 45, 201-206.

IASP. Pharmacological Management of Neuropathic Pain. *Pain*. Clinical updates, 2010, 18, 1-8.

Ishikawa, S; Matsunaga, K; Nakanishi, R; Kawahira, K; Murayama, N; Tsuji, S; et al. Effect of theta burst stimulation over the human sensorimotor cortex on motor and somatosensory evoked potentials. *Clin Neurophysiol*, 2007, 118, 1033-1043.

Jensen, TS; Backonja, MM; Hernandez Jimenez, S; Tesfaye, S; Valensi, P; Ziegler, D. New perspectives on the management of diabetic peripheral neuropathic pain. *Diab Vasc Dis Res*, 2006, 3, 108-119.

Jette, F; Cote, I; Meziane, HB; Mercier, C. Effect of single-session repetitive transcranial magnetic stimulation applied over the hand versus leg motor area on pain after spinal cord injury. *Neurorehabil Neural Repair*, 2013, 27, 636-643.

Jung, SH; Shin, JE; Jeong, YS; Shin, HI. Changes in motor cortical excitability induced by high-frequency repetitive transcranial magnetic stimulation of different stimulation durations. Clin Neurophysiol, 2008, 119, 71-79.

Kang, BS; Shin, HI; Bang, MS. Effect of repetitive transcranial magnetic stimulation over the hand motor cortical area on central pain after spinal cord injury. *Arch Phys Med Rehabil*, 2009, 90, 1766-1771.

Khedr, EM; Gilio, F; Rothwell, J. Effects of low frequency and low intensity repetitive paired pulse stimulation of the primary motor cortex. *Clin Neurophysiol*, 2004, 115, 1259-1263.

Kim, JY; Choi, GS; Cho, YW; Cho, H; Hwang, SJ; Ahn, SH. Attenuation of spinal cord injury-induced astroglial and microglial activation by repetitive transcranial magnetic stimulation in rats. *J Korean Med Sci*, 2013, 28, 295-299.

Kim, YJ; Ku, J; Kim, HJ; Im, DJ; Lee, HS; Han, KA; et al. Randomized, sham controlled trial of transcranial direct current stimulation for painful diabetic polyneuropathy. *Ann Rehabil Med*, 2014, 37, 766-776.

Knotkova, H; Portenoy, RK; Cruciani, RA. Transcranial direct current stimulation (tDCS) relieved itching in a patient with chronic neuropathic pain. *Clin J Pain*, 2013, 29, 621-622.

Kodama, M; Aono, K; Masakado, Y. Changes in sensory functions after low-frequency repetitive transcranial magnetic stimulation over the motor cortex. *Tokai J Exp Clin Med*, 2009, 34, 122-129.

Kumru, H; Soler, D; Vidal, J; Navarro, X; Tormos, JM; Pascual-Leone, A; et al. The effects of transcranial direct current stimulation with visual illusion in neuropathic pain due to spinal cord injury: an evoked potentials and quantitative thermal testing study. *Eur J Pain*, 2012, 17, 55-66.

Kumru, H; Soto, O; Casanova, J; Valls-Sole, J. Motor cortex excitability changes during imagery of simple reaction time. *Exp Brain Res*, 2008, 189, 373-378.

Kuo, MF; Grosch, J; Fregni, F; Paulus, W; Nitsche, MA. Focusing effect of acetylcholine on neuroplasticity in the human motor cortex. *J Neurosci*, 2007, 27, 14442-14447.

Kuo, MF; Paulus, W; Nitsche, MA. Boosting focally-induced brain plasticity by dopamine. Cereb Cortex, 2008, 18, 648-651.

Lalo, E; Gilbertson, T; Doyle, L; Di Lazzaro, V; Cioni, B; Brown, P. Phasic increases in cortical beta activity are associated with alterations in sensory processing in the human. *Exp Brain Res*, 2007, 177, 137-145.

Lang, N; Siebner, HR; Ernst, D; Nitsche, MA; Paulus, W; Lemon, RN; et al. Preconditioning with transcranial direct current stimulation sensitizes the motor cortex to rapid-rate transcranial magnetic stimulation and controls the direction of after-effects. *Biol Psychiatry*, 2004, 56, 634-639.

Lang, N; Siebner, HR; Ward, NS; Lee, L; Nitsche, MA; Paulus, W; et al. How does transcranial DC stimulation of the primary motor cortex alter regional neuronal activity in the human brain? *Eur J Neurosci*, 2005, 22, 495-504.

Lee, MC; Zambreanu, L; Menon, DK; Tracey, I. Identifying brain activity specifically related to the maintenance and perceptual consequence of central sensitization in humans. *J Neurosci*, 2008, 28, 11642-11649.

Lefaucheur, JP; Ayache, SS; Sorel, M; Farhat, WH; Zouari, HG; Ciampi de Andrade, D; et al. Analgesic effects of repetitive transcranial magnetic stimulation of the motor cortex in neuropathic pain: influence of theta burst stimulation priming. *Eur J Pain*, 2012, 16, 1403-1413.

Lefaucheur, JP; Drouot, X; Menard-Lefaucheur, I; Keravel, Y; Nguyen, JP. Motor cortex rTMS restores defective intracortical inhibition in chronic neuropathic pain. *Neurology*, 2006, 67, 1568-1574.

Lefaucheur, JP; Drouot, X; Menard-Lefaucheur, I; Keravel, Y; Nguyen, JP. Motor cortex rTMS in chronic neuropathic pain: pain relief is associated with thermal sensory perception improvement. *J Neurol Neurosurg Psychiatry*, 2008, 79, 1044-1049.

Leung, A; Donohue, M; Xu, R; Lee, R; Lefaucheur, JP; Khedr, EM; et al. rTMS for suppressing neuropathic pain: a meta-analysis. *J Pain*, 2009, 10, 1205-1216.

Liebetanz, D; Nitsche, MA; Tergau, F; Paulus, W. Pharmacological approach to the mechanisms of transcranial DC-stimulation-induced after-effects of human motor cortex excitability. *Brain*, 2002, 125, 2238-2247.

Maeda, F; Keenan, JP; Tormos, JM; Topka, H; Pascual-Leone, A. Modulation of corticospinal excitability by repetitive transcranial magnetic stimulation. *Clin Neurophysiol*, 2000, 111, 800-805.

Maeoka, H; Matsuo, A; Hiyamizu, M; Morioka, S; Ando, H. Influence of transcranial direct current stimulation of the dorsolateral prefrontal cortex on pain related emotions: a study using electroencephalographic power spectrum analysis. *Neurosci Lett*, 2012, 512, 12-16.

Martin, L; Borckardt, JJ; Reeves, ST; Frohman, H; Beam, W; Nahas, Z; et al. A pilot functional MRI study of the effects of prefrontal rTMS on pain perception. Pain Med, 2013, 14, 999-1009.

Matsumura, Y; Hirayama, T; Yamamoto, T. Comparison between pharmacologic evaluation and repetitive transcranial magnetic stimulation-induced analgesia in poststroke pain patients. *Neuromodulation*, 2013, 16, 349-354; discussion 354.

Medeiros, LF; de Souza, IC; Vidor, LP; de Souza, A; Deitos, A; Volz, MS; et al. Neurobiological effects of transcranial direct current stimulation: a review. *Front Psychiatry*, 2013, 3, 110.

Migita, K; Uozumi, T; Arita, K; Monden, S. Transcranial magnetic coil stimulation of motor cortex in patients with central pain. *Neurosurgery*, 1995, 36, 1037-1039; discussion 1039-1040.

Moisset, X; Villain, N; Ducreux, D; Serrie, A; Cunin, G; Valade, D; et al. Functional brain imaging of trigeminal neuralgia. *Eur J Pain*, 2011, 15, 124-131.

Moloney, TM; Witney, AG. Transcranial direct current stimulation (tDCS) priming of 1Hz repetitive transcranial magnetic stimulation (rTMS) modulates experimental pain thresholds. *Neurosci Lett*, 2012, 534, 289-294.

Monte-Silva, K; Kuo, MF; Liebetanz, D; Paulus, W; Nitsche, MA. Shaping the optimal repetition interval for cathodal transcranial direct current stimulation (tDCS). *J Neurophysiol*, 2010, 103, 1735-1740.

Monte-Silva, K; Kuo, MF; Thirugnanasambandam, N; Liebetanz, D; Paulus, W; Nitsche, MA. Dose-dependent inverted U-shaped effect of dopamine (D2-like) receptor activation on focal and nonfocal plasticity in humans. *J Neurosci*, 2009, 29, 6124-6131.

Moont, R; Crispel, Y; Lev, R; Pud, D; Yarnitsky, D. Temporal changes in cortical activation during conditioned pain modulation (CPM), a LORETA study. *Pain*, 2011, 152, 1469-1477.

Mori, F; Codeca, C; Kusayanagi, H; Monteleone, F; Buttari, F; Fiore, S; et al. Effects of anodal transcranial direct current stimulation on chronic neuropathic pain in patients with multiple sclerosis. *J Pain*, 2009, 11, 436-442.

Murakami, T; Sakuma, K; Nomura, T; Nakashima, K; Hashimoto, I. High-frequency oscillations change in parallel with short-interval intracortical inhibition after theta burst magnetic stimulation. *Clin Neurophysiol*, 2008, 119, 301-308.

Nahmias, F; Debes, C; de Andrade, DC; Mhalla, A; Bouhassira, D. Diffuse analgesic effects of unilateral repetitive transcranial magnetic stimulation (rTMS) in healthy volunteers. *Pain*, 2009, 147, 224-232.

NICE (2013). Neuropathic pain – pharmacological management. p. 41.

Nitsche, MA; Kuo, MF; Karrasch, R; Wachter, B; Liebetanz, D; Paulus, W. Serotonin affects transcranial direct current-induced neuroplasticity in humans. *Biol Psychiatry*, 2009, 66, 503-508.

Nitsche, MA; Liebetanz, D; Tergau, F; Paulus, W. [Modulation of cortical excitability by transcranial direct current stimulation]. *Nervenarzt*, 2002, 73, 332-335.

Nitsche, MA; Niehaus, L; Hoffmann, KT; Hengst, S; Liebetanz, D; Paulus, W; et al. MRI study of human brain exposed to weak direct current stimulation of the frontal cortex. *Clin Neurophysiol*, 2004, 115, 2419-2423.

Nitsche, MA; Seeber, A; Frommann, K; Klein, CC; Rochford, C; Nitsche, MS; et al. Modulating parameters of excitability during and after transcranial direct current stimulation of the human motor cortex. *J Physiol*, 2005, 568, 291-303.

Nizard, J; Lefaucheur, JP; Helbert, M; de Chauvigny, E; Nguyen, JP. Non-invasive stimulation therapies for the treatment of refractory pain. *Discov Med*, 2012, 14, 21-31.

Norrbrink Budh, C; Lund, I; Ertzgaard, P; Holtz, A; Hultling, C; Levi, R; et al. Pain in a Swedish spinal cord injury population. *Clin Rehabil*, 2003, 17, 685-690.

O'Connell, NE; Wand, BM; Marston, L; Spencer, S; Desouza, LH. Non-invasive brain stimulation techniques for chronic pain. A report of a Cochrane systematic review and meta-analysis. *Eur J Phys Rehabil Med*, 2011, 47, 309-326.

Oberman, L; Edwards, D; Eldaief, M; Pascual-Leone, A. Safety of theta burst transcranial magnetic stimulation: a systematic review of the literature. *J Clin Neurophysiol*, 2012, 28, 67-74.

Ohn, SH; Chang, WH; Park, CH; Kim, ST; Lee, JI; Pascual-Leone, A; et al. Neural correlates of the antinociceptive effects of repetitive transcranial magnetic stimulation on central pain after stroke. *Neurorehabil Neural Repair*, 2012, 26, 344-352.

Onesti, E; Gabriele, M; Cambieri, C; Ceccanti, M; Raccah, R; Di Stefano, G; et al. H-coil repetitive transcranial magnetic stimulation for pain relief in patients with diabetic neuropathy. *Eur J Pain*, 2013, 17, 1347-1356.

Palm, U; Keeser, D; Schiller, C; Fintescu, Z; Nitsche, M; Reisinger, E et al. Skin lesions after treatment with transcranial direct current stimulation (tDCS). *Brain Stimul*, 2008, 1, 386-387.

Pascual-Leone, A; Amedi, A; Fregni, F; Merabet, LB. The plastic human brain cortex. *Annu Rev Neurosci*, 2005, 28, 377-401.

Pascual-Leone, A; Houser, CM; Reese, K; Shotland, LI; Grafman, J; Sato, S et al. Safety of rapid-rate transcranial magnetic stimulation in normal volunteers. Electroencephalogr *Clin Neurophysiol*, 1993, 89, 120-130.

Pascual-Leone, A; Tormos, JM; Keenan, J; Tarazona, F; Canete, C; Catala, MD. Study and modulation of human cortical excitability with transcranial magnetic stimulation. *J Clin Neurophysiol*, 1998, 15, 333-343.

Pell, GS; Roth, Y; Zangen, A. Modulation of cortical excitability induced by repetitive transcranial magnetic stimulation: influence of timing and geometrical parameters and underlying mechanisms. *Prog Neurobiol*, 2011, 93, 59-98.

Plow, EB; Pascual-Leone, A; Machado, A. Brain stimulation in the treatment of chronic neuropathic and non-cancerous pain. *J Pain*, 2012, 13, 411-424.

Pogosyan, A; Gaynor, LD; Eusebio, A; Brown, P. Boosting cortical activity at Beta-band frequencies slows movement in humans. *Curr Biol*, 2009, 19, 1637-1641.

Poreisz, C; Antal, A; Boros, K; Brepohl, N; Csifcsak, G; Paulus, W. Attenuation of N2 amplitude of laser-evoked potentials by theta burst stimulation of primary somatosensory cortex. *Exp Brain Res*, 2008, 185, 611-621.

Poreisz, C; Boros, K; Antal, A; Paulus, W. Safety aspects of transcranial direct current stimulation concerning healthy subjects and patients. *Brain Res Bull*, 2007, 72, 208-214.

Reidler, JS; Mendonca, ME; Santana, MB; Wang, X; Lenkinski, R; Motta, AF et al. Effects of motor cortex modulation and descending inhibitory systems on pain thresholds in healthy subjects. *J Pain*, 2012, 13, 450-458.

Rossi, S; Hallett, M; Rossini, PM; Pascual-Leone, A. Safety, ethical considerations, and application guidelines for the use of transcranial magnetic stimulation in clinical practice and research. *Clin Neurophysiol*, 2009, 120, 2008-2039.

Rothkegel, H; Sommer, M; Paulus, W. Breaks during 5Hz rTMS are essential for facilitatory after effects. *Clin Neurophysiol*, 2010, 121, 426-430.

Sakas, DE; Panourias, IG; Simpson, BA; Krames, ES. An introduction to operative neuromodulation and functional neuroprosthetics, the new frontiers of clinical neuroscience and biotechnology. *Acta Neurochir Suppl*, 2007, 97, 3-10.

Sampson, SM; Kung, S; McAlpine, DE; Sandroni, P. The use of slow-frequency prefrontal repetitive transcranial magnetic stimulation in refractory neuropathic pain. *J ECT*, 2011, 27, 33-37.

Schabrun, SM; Chipchase, LS; Zipf, N; Thickbroom, GW; Hodges, PW. Interaction between simultaneously applied neuromodulatory interventions in humans. *Brain Stimul*, 2012, 6, 624-630.

Schmader, KE. Epidemiology and impact on quality of life of postherpetic neuralgia and painful diabetic neuropathy. Clin J Pain, 2002, 18, 350-354.

Shipton, E. Post-surgical neuropathic pain. *ANZ J Surg*, 2008, 78, 548-555.

Siddall, PJ; McClelland, JM;Rutkowski, SB; Cousins, MJ. A longitudinal study of the prevalence and characteristics of pain in the first 5 years following spinal cord injury. *Pain*, 2003, 103, 249-257.

Siebner, HR; Lang, N; Rizzo, V; Nitsche, MA; Paulus, W; Lemon, RN; Rothwell, JC. Preconditioning of low-frequency repetitive transcranial magnetic stimulation with transcranial direct current stimulation: evidence for homeostatic plasticity in the human motor cortex. *J Neurosci*, 2004, 24, 3379-3385.

Sokal, P; Sokal, K. The neuromodulative role of earthing. *Med Hypotheses*, 2011, 77, 824-826.

Soler, MD; Kumru, H; Pelayo, R; Vidal, J; Tormos, JM; Fregni, F; et al. Effectiveness of transcranial direct current stimulation and visual illusion on neuropathic pain in spinal cord injury. *Brain*, 2010, 133, 2565-2577.

Soler, MD; Sauri-Ruiz, J; Curcoll-Gallemi, ML; Benito-Penalva, J; Opisso-Salleras, E; Chamarro-Lusar, A; Vidal-Samso, J. [Characteristics of chronic neuropathic pain and their relationship with psychological well-being in spinal cord injury patients]. *Rev Neurol*, 2007, 44, 3-9.

Sommer, M; Norden, C; Schmack, L; Rothkegel, H; Lang, N; Paulus, W. Opposite optimal current flow directions for induction of neuroplasticity and excitation threshold in the human motor cortex. *Brain Stimul*, 2013, 6, 363-370.

Speer, AM; Kimbrell, TA; Wassermann, EM; D Repella J.; Willis, MW; Herscovitch, P; et al. Opposite effects of high and low frequency rTMS on regional brain activity in depressed patients. *Biol Psychiatry*, 2000, 48, 1133-1141.

Stagg, CJ; Bachtiar, V; Amadi, U; Gudberg, CA; Ilie, AS; Sampaio-Baptista, C; et al. Local GABA concentration is related to network-level resting functional connectivity. *Elife*, 2014, 3, e01465.

Stagg, CJ; Lin, RL; Mezue, M; Segerdahl, A; Kong, Y; Xie, J; et al. Widespread modulation of cerebral perfusion induced during and after transcranial direct current stimulation applied to the left dorsolateral prefrontal cortex. *J Neurosci*, 2013, 33, 11425-11431.

Stanwell, P; Siddall, P; Keshava, N; Cocuzzo, D; Ramadan, S; Lin, A; et al. Neuro magnetic resonance spectroscopy using wavelet decomposition and statistical testing identifies biochemical changes in people with spinal cord injury and pain. *Neuroimage*, 2010, 53, 544-552.

Taylor, JJ; Borckardt, JJ; George, MS. Endogenous opioids mediate left dorsolateral prefrontal cortex rTMS-induced analgesia. *Pain*, 2012, 153, 1219-1225.

Topper, R; Foltys, H; Meister, IG; Sparing, R; Boroojerdi, B. Repetitive transcranial magnetic stimulation of the parietal cortex transiently ameliorates phantom limb pain-like syndrome. *Clin Neurophysiol*, 2003, 114, 1521-1530.

Treister, R; Lang, M; Klein, MM; Oaklander, AL. Non-invasive Transcranial Magnetic Stimulation (TMS) of the Motor Cortex for Neuropathic Pain-At the Tipping Point? *Rambam Maimonides Med J*, 2013, 4, e0023.

Tsubokawa, T; Katayama, Y; Yamamoto, T; Hirayama, T; Koyama, S. Chronic motor cortex stimulation for the treatment of central pain. *Acta Neurochir Suppl (Wien)*, 1991, 52, 137-139.

Valero-Cabre, A; Pascual-Leone, A; Rushmore, RJ. Cumulative sessions of repetitive transcranial magnetic stimulation (rTMS) build up facilitation to subsequent TMS-mediated behavioural disruptions. *Eur J Neurosci*, 2008, 27, 765-774.

Vaseghi, B; Zoghi, M; Jaberzadeh, S. Does anodal transcranial direct current stimulation modulate sensory perception and pain? A meta-analysis study. *Clin Neurophysiol*, 2014.

Villamar, MF; Volz, MS; Bikson, M; Datta, A; Dasilva, AF; Fregni, F. Technique and considerations in the use of 4x1 ring high-definition transcranial direct current stimulation (HD-tDCS). *J Vis Exp*, 2013, e50309.

Wassermann, EM; Wedegaertner, FR; Ziemann, U; George, MS; Chen, R. Crossed reduction of human motor cortex excitability by 1-Hz transcranial magnetic stimulation. *Neurosci Lett*, 1998, 250, 141-144.

Widerstrom-Noga, E; Pattany, PM; Cruz-Almeida, Y; Felix, ER; Perez, S; Cardenas, DD et al. Metabolite concentrations in the anterior cingulate cortex predict high neuropathic pain impact after spinal cord injury. *Pain*, 2013, 154, 204-212.

Wrigley, PJ; Gustin, SM; McIndoe, LN; Chakiath, RJ; Henderson, LA; Siddall, PJ. Longstanding neuropathic pain after spinal cord injury is refractory to transcranial direct current stimulation: a randomized controlled trial. *Pain*, 2013, 154, 2178-2184.

Yoo, WK; You, SH; Ko, MH; Tae Kim, S; Park, CH; Park, JW; et al. High frequency rTMS modulation of the sensorimotor networks: behavioral changes and fMRI correlates. *Neuroimage*, 2008, 39, 1886-1895.

Yoon, EJ; Kim, YK; Kim, HR; Kim, SE; Lee, Y; Shin, HI. Transcranial direct current stimulation to lessen neuropathic pain after spinal cord injury: a mechanistic PET study. *Neurorehabil Neural Repair*, 2013, 28, 250-259.

Zaghi, S; Heine, N; Fregni, F. Brain stimulation for the treatment of pain: A review of costs, clinical effects, and mechanisms of treatment for three different central neuromodulatory approaches. *J Pain Manag*, 2009, 2, 339-352.

In: Neuropathic Pain
Editor: Alyssa L. Rider
ISBN: 978-1-63321-963-2

Chapter 2

Neuropathic Pain in Spinal Cord Injury

Timothy R. Cushing, MD[1,*], Sujin Lee, MD[2,†], Maya Hatch, PhD[3,‡], Sophia Chun, MD[4,§], and Eric Chang, MD[5,‖]

[1]Department of Physical Medicine and Rehabilitation, University of California, Los Angeles, US
[2]Department of Physical Medicine and Rehabilitation, University of California, Sue and Bill Gross Stem Cell Center, Irvine, CA, US
[3]Reeve-Irvine Research Center for Spinal Cord Injury, University of California, Irvine, CA, US
[4]Veterans Affairs Long Beach Healthcare System, Department of Physical Medicine and Rehabilitation, Long Beach, CA, US
[5]Department of Physical Medicine and Rehabilitation, Department of Neurosurgery, Department of Orthopedics, Reeve-Irvine Research Center for Spinal Cord Injury, University of California, Irvine, CA, US

[*] Timothy R. Cushing, MD. E-mail: momentim@gmail.com.
[†] Sujin Lee, MD. E-mail: sujinl3@uci.edu.
[‡] Maya Hatch, PhD. E-mail: hatchm@uci.edu.
[§] Sophia Chun, MD. E-mail: Sophia.chun@va.gov.
[‖] Eric Chang, MD. E-mail: Changey1@uci.edu.

Abstract

Pain is a common complication in patients following spinal cord injury (SCI), with studies demonstrating up to 80% of patients reporting some form of pain in the years after their injury. Pain can be divided into multiple different subtypes including nociceptive, neuropathic, and psychogenic. Neuropathic pain, and more specifically central neuropathic pain, makes up a substantial percentage of all pain symptoms in patients with SCI. Given the high prevalence of central neuropathic pain in patients with SCI, proper identification and treatment is imperative. Indeed, identification of pain subtypes is a vital step toward determining appropriate treatment, and once determined, a variety of treatment measures can be undertaken. Medications commonly utilized to treat neuropathic pain include anticonvulsants, tricyclic antidepressants, antispastic agents, and opioids. Non-pharmacologic treatment strategies include spinal cord stimulation, physical therapy, physical modalities, psychological interventions, and acupuncture. Additionally, intrathecal delivery of certain medications have become increasingly popular and been shown to significantly reduce neuropathic pain, while causing fewer systemic side effects than oral drugs in patients with SCI. Despite all of the available treatment options and ongoing advances in the field of SCI medicine, providing adequate treatment of central neuropathic pain after SCI continues to be challenging. Management of central neuropathic pain, as with other forms of chronic pain, is complex and often requires a multifaceted and integrative approach. It is therefore extremely important for clinicians to have a good understanding of how central neuropathic pain arises, as well all the available and appropriate treatment options for patients displaying this sort of pain.

In this chapter we will discuss the pathophysiology, identification, and treatment options for patients with SCI displaying central neuropathic pain, giving recommendations where appropriate. We hope that this will not only provide a better understanding of central neuropathic pain for physicians in various subspecialties, but that it will also help guide future research on this important subject.

Introduction

Pain is a common problem in people with spinal cord injury (SCI). Although there is some variation among studies of the prevalence of pain after SCI, approximately 65 to 85% of patients will experience pain, and about a third of this group will suffer from severe pain [1]. Although severe disabling pain exists in the minority of patients with SCI, many more suffer significant decrement in cognitive, physical, and emotional functionality due to the effects of pain [2]. Moreover, about 30-40% of patients with SCI suffer from neuropathic pain due to lesions of nervous structures [3].

Of all the post-injury complications in patients with SCI, pain is one of the most difficult conditions to treat [4] The fundamental problem is that pain in SCI is often complex and multifactorial, and tends to be refractory to the treatments that are currently available. The management of pain requires specific approaches that may not be familiar to physicians who do not routinely manage chronic pain or post-SCI patients. This can result in poor outcomes and reduced quality of life in patients living with SCI.

The goals of this chapter are to provide an understanding of the different types of pain after spinal cord injury, and to provide an in-depth discussion specifically about neuropathic pain in this patient population. We will examine pertinent clinical findings in neuropathic pain, and review multiple clinical tools, which may be of use to physicians attempting to diagnose neuropathic pain. Furthermore, we will investigate the pathophysiology, and potential treatment options for neuropathic pain in patients with SCI.

Pain-Related Terminology, Taxonomy, Definitions, and Clinical Assessment Tools

In order to develop an in-depth understanding of pain experienced in patients with SCI, it is crucial to clarify the different types of pain that can be present in these patients. It also is imperative to discuss pain in relation to level of SCI, which is a phenomenon unique to this population of patients.

Furthermore, we will explore various clinical tools, and pain classification systems that have been developed to assist health-care professionals in the diagnosis of specific types of pain.

There are various ways that pain can be generated in the body, with many tissues being capable of producing painful sensations. An important distinction to understand is the difference between nociceptive pain and neuropathic pain. Nociceptive pain is defined as pain generated from the activation of nociceptors in peripheral tissues. A nociceptor is a nerve ending specializing in detection of noxious stimuli that result in tissue destruction.

Some examples of noxious stimuli include inflammation, thermal energy, ischemia, and compression. Nociceptors can be found in a number of different tissues, including skin, muscles, tendons, bones, and ligaments.

They typically belong to one of two types of nerve fibers: the thin, unmyelinated, slowly conducting (0.5 to 2 m/s) C fibers; or the medium diameter, sparsely myelinated, rapidly conducting (12 to 30 m/s) Aδ fibers [5]. In an individual with normal pain physiology, the purpose of nociception is to alert the brain to actual or potential tissue damage so that avoidance behavior can be initiated.

Nociceptive pain can be further subdivided into musculoskeletal and visceral pain. Musculoskeletal pain is a common and frequently-experienced form of pain, and is due to trauma or inflammation in bones, joints, muscles, or other connective tissue. It can also arise from mechanical instability, muscle spasms, or overuse syndromes. To diagnose this class of pain, it is necessary for the patient to have at least some preserved sensation where the pain is located, and the patient should be able to accurately localize the pain.

Also, evidence of musculoskeletal pathology underlying the pain must exist [6]. Visceral pain is typically poorly localized, and is the result of activation of nociceptors in the abdominal, thoracic, or pelvic organs and tissues. This is the pain associated with certain diagnoses, as in myocardial infarctions, cholecystitis, and kidney stones, and can be activated by stimuli such as distension, compression, inflammation, and ischemia affecting the visceral organs [6].

In contrast to nociceptive pain, neuropathic pain arises as a direct consequence to a lesion or disease affecting the somatosensory system [7]. In other words, neuropathic pain develops due to injury of the nerves themselves. In addition to SCI, neuropathic pain can be caused by systemic diseases causing widespread nerve damage, (i.e. diabetic neuropathy), focal peripheral nerve entrapments, (i.e. carpal tunnel syndrome, piriformis syndrome), and also at the level of the spinal nerve roots, (i.e. radiculopathy, spinal stenosis). People who experience neuropathic pain frequently characterize the sensations as tingling, burning, electric shock-like, cold, pricking, pins and needles, squeezing, sharp, itchy, and/or shooting [6, 8].

Furthermore, patients with neuropathic pain frequently describe their pain as spontaneous (arising without detectable stimulation), or evoked (an abnormal response to stimuli, such as allodynia, and hyperalgesia) [8].

Another important distinction is the difference between peripheral neuropathic pain and central neuropathic pain. Simply stated, a lesion of the peripheral nerve generates peripheral neuropathic pain. This includes the entire peripheral nervous system, from the spinal nerve roots proximally, to the most distal terminals of the nerves. In contrast, a lesion in the central nervous system, which includes the brain, brainstem, and spinal cord, generates central neuropathic pain. SCI is, by definition, a lesion to the central nervous system. Neuropathic pain after SCI is frequently central in origin, and arises as a direct consequence of a lesion affecting the somatosensory system, in particular affecting the spinothalamocortical pathways [6]. Moreover, especially in cases of SCI due to trauma, there can be widespread tissue damage affecting not only the spinal cord, but also the nerve roots, plexuses, and peripheral nerves - from which peripheral neuropathic pain can also arise.

Neuropathic pain is divided into three sub-tiers based on location of the pain in relation to the neurologic level of injury (NLI). "At-level" neuropathic pain is defined as neuropathic pain from a lesion of the nerve root or the spinal cord this is experienced within the dermatome of the NLI, and/or within three dermatomes below the NLI, and/or one dermatome above the NLI [6]. At-level neuropathic pain can be unilateral or bilateral. If the pain is due to a lesion in the cauda equina, at-level neuropathic pain can be experienced up to six levels below the NLI. At-level neuropathic pain can be radicular in nature, due to the fact that spinal nerve roots in the vicinity of a traumatic SCI often are damaged as well. "Below-level" neuropathic pain refers to pain more than three dermatomes below the dermatome of the NLI [6].

A necessary condition for classifying pain as below-level neuropathic pain is that a lesion must affect the spinal cord, and the pain is believed to be a result of that damage. Below-level pain does not typically follow dermatomal patterns, but rather tends to encompass large regions, such as one or both feet, legs, buttocks, or the entire body below the NLI. The third sub-tier is "other" neuropathic pain, which refers to neuropathic pain at any level that is not thought to be directly related to SCI itself [6].

Some examples of other neuropathic pain include upper-extremity compressive mononeuropathies such as carpal tunnel syndrome in patients with paraplegia, pain from lumbar radiculopathy, or diabetic polyneuropathy.

In general, pain assessment in patients with SCI is complex, and requires a combination of standard general pain measures, as well as more specific questions unique to different etiologies of pain, which arise from unique pathological mechanisms. Determination of the NLI is an important step for the clinician to take prior to assessing pain in a patient with SCI. Once NLI is understood, the patient should describe the location, quality, distribution, periodicity, intensity, and duration of the pain, as well as aggravating or alleviating factors. A comprehensive and detailed pain history should include onset of pain, circumstances under which it arose, past treatments attempted, and evolution of the pain over time [9]. After this detailed pain history is obtained, pain evaluation tools and assessments can be properly performed.

Clinicians currently have several pain evaluation tools to establish an objective assessment of central neuropathic pain.

Currently one tool exists which is specific to neuropathic pain after SCI, the Spinal Cord Injury Pain Instrument (SCIPI). This tool was shown to have good sensitivity, specificity and diagnostic accuracy in a SCI population in a recent preliminary validation study [10].

Further study is required before this tool can be universally adopted. However, multiple other instruments are currently available. Common tools to measure pain quantity include the Visual Analog Scale (VAS), the Numeric Rating Scale (NRS), or the Visual Rating Scale (VRS).

Assessment tools specific to central neuropathic pain include the Neuropathic Pain Scale (NPS), the Neuropathic Pain Symptom Inventory, and the Leeds Assessment of Neuropathic Signs and Symptoms [11].

The NPS is a self-administered, multidimensional assessment tool using descriptive terms of pain, such as "sharp, hot, dull, cold, sensitive, itchy, surface, and deep". The Neuropathic Pain Symptom Inventory is a 12-part, self-administered questionnaire evaluating different aspects of the patient's experience of neuropathic pain, such as pain quality, severity of attacks of pain, frequency of symptoms, evoked nature of pain, and abnormal sensations [12]. The self-completed Leeds Assessment of Neuropathic Signs and Symptoms was the first questionnaire developed to obtain a diagnosis of neuropathic pain.

It appears to have the most empirical data showing that it correctly distinguishes neuropathic pain from other types of pain among those with mixed chronic pain. The NPS has the most empirical support as a measure of treatment outcome, although a new measuring instrument, the Pain Quality Assessment Scale, that includes the NPS may prove to be more useful because it incorporates additional pain descriptors not found in the NPS [13].

Future assessment tools and scales will need to be developed to accurately manage and treat patients with central neuropathic pain from SCI. Scales that include patient self-assessment and logarithm-based questions may help capture a patient's pain complaints more accurately than current models. Moreover, as treatments for central neuropathic pain are attempted (as will be discussed below), it will be useful for clinicians to consistently re-evaluate patients with the same, or multiple, assessment tools in order to uncover subtle differences in symptoms which may not be readily apparent with less detailed questionnaires.

Pathophysiology of Neuropathic Pain in SCI

The pathophysiology of neuropathic pain in patients with SCI is a complex and multifactorial phenomenon that is initiated at the time of the injury itself, and is further complicated by secondary neuronal changes and adaptations that develop months to years later.

These changes not only involve the injured segment of spinal cord, but also can be found in remote neural structures, well above, and below the level of injury. The widespread and multifactorial features of damage and physiological changes in SCI may explain why neuropathic pain associated with SCI can be so difficult to treat.

Damage to the nervous system in cases of SCI can be divided into two broad mechanisms: the primary and secondary mechanisms. The primary mechanism is the initial mechanical damage, which causes an insult to the spinal cord itself. More than 70% of SCI are from trauma and morphological changes (fracture, dislocation, instability, disc herniation, ligamentous disruption) in the bony spinal column, which also impinge upon and damage the spinal cord [14]. Primary injury to the spinal cord has four morphologic types: impact plus persistent compression, impact with transient compression, distraction, or transection [15].

The initial impact (primary mechanism) leads to immediate hemorrhage, shearing of axons, edema, vasospasm, plasma membrane compromise, and cell death at the impact site. This is followed by the development of secondary mechanisms, which commence within minutes of SCI and can continue to cause damage to neural structures months later. There are at least 25 unique processes that compose the secondary mechanism in SCI.

These processes include inflammation, changes in immune function, plasma membrane disruption, loss of ionic homeostasis, excitotoxicity, free-radical production, apoptosis, scar formation, and more [15].

The above-mentioned events have an interdependent relationship and collectively create an environment responsible for changing the functional and physiological state of spinal sensory neurons that may lead to expression of different clinical conditions such as allodynia, hyperalgesia, and spontaneous pain [16]. The anatomical and functional changes that occur in the nervous system after SCI can contribute to hyperexcitability of higher neurons as well as disinhibition and imbalance of the pathway [16]. Indeed, previous studies have shown that deafferentation of peripheral nerves may cause denervation hyperexcitability of more proximal neurons, and partial lesions may cause disinhibition or an imbalance in between pathways [17].

Furthermore, it should be noted that changes in regional anatomical and connectivity within the brain itself have been documented in patients with persistent neuropathic pain after SCI [18]. This data further illustrates the far-reaching affects that SCI can have within the nervous system.

Treatment of Neuropathic Pain in SCI

There is a broad range of pharmacological and non-pharmacological treatments that can be employed in the treatment of neuropathic pain in patients with SCI. As will be further discussed, these various treatments aim to address the abnormalities occurring at the spinal, brain, and peripheral level. Prior to starting medications, it is always important to determine that neuropathic pain is the most likely etiology of the patient's discomfort. Before pharmacologic agents are prescribed, it is important to confirm that proper etiologic factors such as correct seating position, proper transferring technique, and correct application and use of bracing and other assistive equipment are addressed. While many of the medications for neuropathic pain are frequently well-tolerated, most of them can have uncomfortable, or even harmful side-effects for patients. Caution must always be exercised when starting or increasing the dose of any such medication.

Similarly, spinal injections, placement of intrathecal pumps, and surgeries expose patients to further risks. As such, practitioners must be prepared to recognize, and manage potential side-effects and adverse events associated with these medications and procedures.

1. Antiepileptics

Antiepileptic drugs are widely used in the treatment of neuropathic pain in patients with SCI. While drugs from this category have been used for many years to treat neuropathic pain, some other the newer members of this class have emerged as popular options, and often as first-line treatments for neuropathic pain in SCI [19]. Gabapentin and pregabalin have replaced older agents such as valproate, carbemazepine, and phenytoin.

These older agents can still be used, but their administration is complicated by higher risk of serious side effects, and often a need to monitor labs for toxicity. Antiepileptics have pharmacologic effect on various pathophysiologic mechanisms that may be involved in neuropathic pain.

Mechanisms of action of this medication class include sodium and calcium channel modulation, and suppression of neuronal hyperexcitability via GABA transmission [20].

Pregabalin is currently approved for the treatment of neuropathic pain in more than 100 countries. In the United States, it has been FDA approved for the treatment of pain due to diabetic peripheral neuropathy, postherpetic neuralgia, fibromyalgia, and as of 2012, neuropathic pain related to SCI. Along with gabapentin, it is a ligand of the alpha(2)-delta subunit of voltage-gated calcium channel.

Several studies have now demonstrated efficacy of pregabalin over placebo, in patients with neuropathic pain associated with SCI [21, 22]. A recent study by Martinez, et al. also demonstrated the analgesic effects of intranasal and intrathecal pregabalin administration in rats in a hypersensitive state caused by spinal nerve ligation and diabetic peripheral neuropathy models [23]. Side effects commonly associated with pregabalin include somnolence, dizziness, peripheral edema, dry mouth, fatigue, and blurred vision. However, these side effects are infrequently severe enough to cause the patient to discontinue the medication [22].

This suggests that the medication is generally well tolerated, and that the analgesic benefits frequently outweigh the adverse effects. Practitioners should be aware that reduced dosing is required in patients with renal insufficiency whose creatinine clearance falls below 60 mL/min. One rare but serious side effect that prescribers should be aware of is that pregabalin may cause suicidal thoughts or actions in a very small percentage of patients.

Despite these issues, pregabalin may be the best medication currently available for SCI patients with neuropathic pain.

Gabapentin is another member of newer generation of antiepileptic medications that is widely used in neuropathic pain. Various studies have been conducted to examine the effectiveness of gabapentin in the treatment of neuropathic pain after SCI. The results have not been uniformly positive or convincing [19]. However, a recent systematic review was able to demonstrate large effect sizes for neuropathic pain improvement with gabapentin monotherapy in patients with SCI [24].

Furthermore, like pregabalin, gabapentin has an improved safety profile over the older antiepileptic agents. Common adverse reactions of gabapentin are also similar to those of pregabalin, including dizziness, drowsiness, fatigue, ataxia, and peripheral edema. Caution must be exercised in patients with renal insufficiency when dosing gabapentin, and dosing adjustments must be made once creatinine clearance falls below 60 mL/min.

First generation anticonvulsants include phenytoin and carbemazepine, which exert membrane-stabilizing effects by blocking neuronal sodium channels. These medications, along with other older-generation anti-epileptics (phenobarbital and valproic acid) have fallen out of common use for the treatment of neuropathic pain secondary to their unfavorable metabolic and interaction profiles. The need for constant monitoring while on these medications make them less practical in the outpatient chronic pain management practice when more favorable side effect profile medications are available. Moreover, there is limited evidence that any of these medications can exert significant, lasting benefit in neuropathic pain after SCI [20].

However, blockade of sodium channels around the time of SCI may reduce secondary neuronal damage, and increase recovery from trauma. A number of animal studies have demonstrated the protective effects of phenytoin on spinal neural structures, when administered at or around the time of spinal cord injury [25, 26]. This suggests that a possible role for sodium channel blockers as a potential therapy to prevent excitotoxic spread of neuronal damage in the timeframe around acute SCI.

Lamotrigine blocks voltage-dependent sodium channels, N-type calcium channels, and inhibits glutamate release [27]. Prior to the emergence of recent studies demonstrating efficacy of pregabalin and gabapentin, lamotrigine was considered a first-line agent in central neuropathic pain [24]. However, a recent Cochrane review on the effect of lamotrigine on neuropathic pain and fibromyalgia reported that there is no convincing evidence of this medication's usefulness in those conditions [28]. However, a randomized controlled trial (RCT) on lamotrigine, for patients with neuropathic pain from SCI, was able to demonstrate a reduction in spontaneous and evoked pain in patients with incomplete SCI only [29]. Caution must be heeded when prescribing lamotrigine in patients with significant hepatic and renal impairment, and those taking other anti-epileptic drugs. In these cases, dose adjustment may be required. The most common adverse effects seen with this medication are rash, headache, dizziness, diplopia, ataxia, somnolence, nausea, and vomiting.

Topiramate is a broad-spectrum anti-convulsant, glutamate receptor antagonist which has been FDA approved to treat epileptic seizures and migraines. This medication has a number of other proposed mechanisms, including GABAergic agonism, and inhibition of voltage-gated sodium and calcium channels. A recent animal study showed that topiramate is effective at reducing loss of neurons and oligodendrocytes when administered shortly after SCI [30]. As previously mentioned for sodium channel blockers such as phenytoin, this data may suggest a role for topiramate in the treatment of acute SCI. Otherwise, the research into the use of topiramate in the treatment of neuropathic pain after SCI is limited, although a number of case studies suggest that topiramate may be an effective treatment in this population [31].

Interestingly, a known side-effect of topiramate is the significant weight loss seen in patients taking this medication [32]. This could confer an additional benefit to SCI patients whose mobility is further restricted by obesity. It should be noted that topiramate requires a careful titration schedule with incremental dose increases performed over weeks.

Dose adjustments is necessary in patients with renal impairments (Cr Cl <70mL/min) and hepatic disease. The most common adverse reactions associated with topiramate include difficulty with memory, fatigue, insomnia, and as previously mentioned, weight loss and anorexia. Patients taking topiramate may also experience parasthesias, which can further complicate the clinical picture in patients with SCI.

2. Tricyclic Antidepressants

Tricyclic antidepressants (TCAs) are hypothesized to exert their effects through the inhibition of the reuptake of sodium and serotonin at the neuronal terminals and through their effects on histamine, muscarinic, and opioid receptors [33]. These medications have been found to be effective in the treatment of a number of chronic pain conditions, including peripheral neuropathy [34]. The analgesic affect produced by TCAs has also been postulated to be caused by increased serotonin in the CNS, thereby inhibiting afferent pain signals [35]. TCAs are generally considered to be first-line treatments in patients with neuropathic pain, along with calcium channel alpha (2)-delta ligands (i.e. pregabalin and gabapentin), SNRIs and topical lidocaine [36]. While these medications tend to be well tolerated, physicians and patients should be aware of various side-effects which are associated with the serotonergic, noradrenergic, and antihistminergic properties of TCAs.

Dizziness, dry mouth, sedation, orthostatic hypotension, blurred vision, gastric distress, urinary retention, and agitation can commonly be seen with use of TCAs. Dosing these medications at night can minimize the interference that these side effects may exert on a patient's daily life.

Patients who are concomitantly taking TCAs with other antidepressants such as selective serotonin reuptake inhibitors (SSRIs), or the codeine analog tramadol are at higher risk of developing serotonin syndrome.

Additionally, TCAs can cause QT prolongation. Practitioners may consider performing an ECG in patients with known cardiac issues or QT prolongation prior to starting this medication.

Amitriptyline is a TCA which has been widely used in the treatment of neuropathic pain. Multiple trials have been conducted, examining the effect of this medication in patients with pain after SCI. One RCT treating a group of people with both neuropathic and musculoskeletal SCI pain found no significant differences in pain intensity, or pain-related disability between groups treated with amitriptyline versus placebo [37]. Another more recent study found amitriptyline to be efficacious in relieving at-level or below-level neuropathic pain, but only in a subgroup of patients with higher scores for depression [38]. Currently, there is not compelling evidence to call for the routine use of TCAs in neuropathic pain due to SCI. However, given that they are relatively well tolerated and safe, this may be a reasonable option for SCI pain, especially in patients with co-morbid depression.

Additionally, nortriptyline and desipramine may be preferable because they typically cause less sedation and have fewer anticholinergic effects.

3. Opioids

Opioids exert their therapeutic effects through modulation of both central and peripheral pain pathways. Opioids interact with specific μ-, κ-, and σ-receptors that block the release of excitatory neurotransmitters such as substance P and glutamate. Opioids also induce neuron hyperpolarization post-synaptically, decreasing synaptic transmission.

It is the μ- receptor that mediates most of the analgesic and respiratory effects. While opioid medications are potent analgesics, their use in both chronic pain and neuropathic pain remains to be controversial due to various physiological, pathological, and psychosocial issues that can arise with their use. In general, opioids are not commonly recommended as first line treatment of patients with SCI and central neuropathic pain [39].

However, one randomized controlled trial using intravenous morphine, and another using alfentanil were able to demonstrate significant reduction in neuropathic pain following SCI [40, 41]. Despite these findings, the evidence is sparse regarding the use of specific oral or transdermal opioids in the treatment of neuropathic pain from SCI. A Cochrane review on the use of opioids in neuropathic pain (non-specific to SCI) originally published in 2006, and updated in 2013 reported that while some studies were able to demonstrate significant efficacy of opioids over placebo in the intermediate term, the use of opioids in chronic neuropathic pain is subject to considerable controversy [42].

The use of chronic opioid analgesic therapy must be approached cautiously due to a range of problems, which include constipation, drowsiness, nausea, dizziness, and vomiting [42]. Other concerning side effects include development of tolerance and need for escalating doses of medication, physical and psychological dependence, development of opioid-induced hyperalgesia, and the possibility of death due to overdose. Moreover, patients using long-term opioids may develop endocrine abnormalities, including decreased testosterone, progesterone, estradiol, and reduced cortisol response to stress [43].

Tramadol is a weak μ-receptor agonist which also has serotonergic and noradrenergic effects. Like other opioid medications, the onset of analgesic action is relatively rapid, but the risk of abuse is lower with tramadol. One RCT performed on patients with at-or-below level neuropathic pain after SCI was able to demonstrate improvement in pain in patients taking tramadol, versus those on placebo [44]. The authors suggest that tramadol may be an option for SCI patients with neuropathic pain which have not responded to gabapentin, pregabalin, or TCAs.

Adverse reactions commonly associated with tramadol include flushing, dizziness, headache, somnolence, pruritis, constipation, nausea, and vomiting.

Tramadol also lowers the seizure threshold, and can contribute to the development of serotonin syndrome when combined with SSRIs, SNRIs, or TCAs. Older patients and those with renal or hepatic impairment should be treated with reduced dosages.

4. Topical Agents

Topical medications offer a key advantage over oral medications due to a lower level of systemic absorption, and by that same token, a much lower risk of developing adverse side effects and drug-drug interactions. Topical agents, in addition to other cutaneously applied treatment such as ice and heat, are useful tools in the approach to both acute and chronic pain. They can provide pain relief in a very localized manner. When used judiciously, topical agents can sometimes supplant the need for scheduled doses of oral medications, which reduces the overall pill burden, and spares the body from potential toxicities of oral medications. Various topical medications are commonly used for pain management, including menthol creams, lidocaine cream and patches, capsaicin, arnica, and topical formulations of NSAIDs and TCAs.

The 5% lidocaine patch has proven efficacious in various neuropathic pain conditions, which allows consideration by many to be a first-line agent [36]. Lidocaine gel (5%) has also shown efficacy in neuropathic pain, and is a less expensive alternative to the patch. This medication can be of most benefit in patients with well-localized neuropathic pain. However, patients with spinal cord injury may suffer from widespread neuropathic pain, thus limiting the use of patches or topical creams. However, this medication has excellent tolerability, with little systemic absorption (it is considered safe to wear up to 3 patches at a time for 12 hours), and the most common side effect is local skin reaction at the site of application. The lack of systemic adverse effects and drug interactions can be especially advantageous in elderly patients and for those in whom polypharmacy is a concern [36].

Capsaicin is another topical medication that may be useful as an adjunctive medication in the treatment of neuropathic pain in SCI. Capsaicin, the pungent agent found in chili peppers, exerts its effect at the vallinoid receptor, which is a detector of noxious heat, and low pH. Capsaicin activates these receptors, which transmits nociceptive information to the central nervous system and releases substance P [45]. This leads eventually to a depletion of substance P and a desensitization period. One small study was able to demonstrate a significant short term (1-2 week) and long term (6 months to >2 years) pain relief in patients with at-level neuropathic pain after SCI [45]. Based on these results and minimal side effects, capsaicin can safely be considered in the treatment of localized radicular pain secondary to SCI, and also may be of use in below-level pain as well.

5. Cannabinoids

Cannabinoid receptors modulate a variety of physiologic processes, including pain, mood, and memory. Cannabinoids have received attention in recent years in part because of preclinical studies that have shown a potential for analgesic effect [46].

Numerous RCTs have been conducted testing the efficacy of cannabinoids on of a variety of chronic pain syndromes. Multiple systematic reviews have found moderate analgesic effect in patients with chronic pain, but questions remain about the long-term safety of cannabinoids [47].

A number of studies have been conducted on the effect of cannabinoids in the treatment of neuropathic pain after SCI. One study comparing dronabinol against an active placebo (diphenhydramine) found no significant difference in relief of below-level neuropathic pain [48]. While other research has shown an improvement in spasticity in patients treated with cannabinoids, this class of medications continues to remain unproven as a reliable analgesic for neuropathic pain following SCI [49]. Cannabinoids tend to be well-tolerated with mild, transient side effects, which most commonly include dry mouth, sedation, dizziness, nausea, and difficulty concentrating [47].

6. Anesthetics

Multiple studies have examined the intravenous administration of various anesthetics in the treatment of neuropathic pain after SCI. Intravenous lidocaine has been found to be effective in the relief of SCI neuropathic pain in a number of studies [50]. The analgesic effect is likely due to lidocaine's action as a blocker of central sodium channels, which reduces neuronal hyperexcitability [50]. The NMDA receptor is another potential target, which can be blocked in order to reduce neuronal hyperexcitability. Ketamine is an antagonist of the NMDA receptor, and has also been shown to be effective on pain after SCI [51].

Despite the findings, the results of these studies are currently of limited clinical utility due to the short-term pain relief provided by these medications, and the practical obstacles of providing long-term parenteral drug delivery.

7. Antispasticity Medications

In general, antispasticity medications have been used in SCI to alleviate spasticity—velocity dependent increases in tone in response to the body's abnormal tonic stretch reflex. However, antispasticity medications, such as baclofen may also be able to exert a significant benefit on central neuropathic pain in patients with SCI. The data remains limited to date, but is suggestive of a future role of antispasticity medications in the management of this problem.

Baclofen is a GABA-B receptor agonist that acts at the level of the spinal cord, and can be administered either orally or intrathecally [52]. Intrathecal baclofen is often the preferred method of administration because it acts directly on the CNS and results in more than 100 times increase in potency delivered at the tissues most responsible for spasticity, with only a fraction of the dose, when compared with oral baclofen [53]. Baclofen's ability to reduce spasticity accounts for its ability to improve musculoskeletal pain. However, multiple studies suggest that it may also have a significant impact on relieving neuropathic pain as well. A small RCT was able to demonstrate a significant reduction in neuropathic burning pain in 6 of 7 subjects treated with intrathecal baclofen [52].

In another study involving 24 patients with SCI, baclofen was effective in reducing pain symptoms in half the patient population [54]. Another recent study demonstrated that intrathecal baclofen was effective in modulating the heat pain perception threshold and heat pain-related evoked potentials in patients with SCI and severe spasticity [55]. Adverse reactions most frequently reported with baclofen include drowsiness, vertigo, dizziness, weakness, slurred speech, and hypotension. Lower doses are advised in elderly patients, as they may be more sensitive to the CNS effects of this medication. An implanted pump commonly delivers intrathecal baclofen, and this is also associated with many potential adverse events from surgical implantation. Other problems that may arise, but are uncommon with the newer technology, are migration, breakage, obstruction, or kinking of the catheter; malfunction of the pump itself; and CSF leakage [56].

8. Use of Combination Pharmacotherapy

A combination drug treatment strategy, in which multiple pain-related mechanisms are engaged, could be more efficacious than single-drug therapy. Addition of a second drug to a pain management regimen could affect the patient in various ways. On one hand, the concern and risk for adverse events is likely to increase with polypharmacy. This is especially the case in the use of drugs in the above-mentioned categories, which commonly have a sedating effect on the CNS. On the other hand, it is possible that by engaging multiple pain mechanisms through the use of medication combination, one could potentially reduce the doses of the individual drugs, thereby minimizing the potential for adverse events [57]. A few clinical studies have been performed examining medication combinations in patients with SCI, which will be discussed here. However, given the paucity of studies performed in this arena, there are no current guidelines or recommendations for multi-drug regimens for neuropathic pain in SCI. One medication combination that was found to have a synergistic analgesic effect was the intrathecal delivery of morphine with clonidine, an α-2 adrenergic agonist [58].

When these medications were given as a mixture, they produced greater at-level, and below-level neuropathic pain relief, than either drug alone. Another combination evaluated in SCI patients with neuropathic pain was the addition of intravenous ketamine to oral gabapentin [59].

This study showed a marked improvement in average pain scores in comparison to the placebo group. Another study performed on patients with neuropathic pain from diabetic neuropathy or post-herpetic neuralgia compared treatment with gabapentin alone against combination treatment with gabapentin and morphine [60]. Gabapentin and morphine combined achieved better analgesia at lower doses than either drug as a single agent.

9. Invasive and Surgical Procedures

Pharmacotherapy is often not sufficient to relieve pain in individuals after SCI. The use of invasive and surgical procedures may be effective in producing more definitive relief. Intrathecal baclofen pumps, as was previously discussed in this chapter, are just one of many invasive measures that can be attempted to relieve neuropathic pain in spinal cord injury. Other procedures that will be discussed in this section include epidural corticosteroid injections, dorsal root entry zone (DREZ) lesioning, implantation of spinal cord stimulators, and other intrathecal drug delivery systems.

Epidural corticosteroid injections have long been established as providing highly effective, although transient pain relief in neuropathic pain secondary to spinal conditions such as radiculopathy and spinal stenosis. This procedure appears to confer the most benefit in SCI when patients have at-level (radicular) neuropathic pain, or when used to treat neuropathic pain from radiculopathies above the level of injury. These findings were demonstrated in a case study [61]. The longevity of the analgesic effect, however, appears to be limited to less than a year, and patients frequently experience return of pain much earlier than that. The use of epidural steroids is also burdened with many risks, due to their potential metabolic, endocrine, immunologic, and psychological side effects. This medication and procedure must be used with caution, or avoided altogether, in patients with underlying diabetes mellitus, osteoporosis, cancer, immunocompromised states, and psychiatric illness. In addition, any procedure involving the spine always carries the risk of further iatrogenic neurologic injury from instrumentation, bleeding, or infection.

Dorsal root entry zone (DREZ) ablation treatments, such as DREZ lesioning and microsurgical DREZotomy are an alternative surgical treatment which can be considered in patients with pain refractory to pharmacological treatment [62]. The DREZ ablation treatments seek to provide pain relief by targeting the nociceptive fibers of the lateral horn of the dorsal rootlet, the medial portion of the Lissauer tract, and the deafferentiated neurons of the dorsal horn [63, 64]. One caveat to the use of this procedure is that it is only considered a treatment option in patients with complete SCI, as patients with incomplete SCI would have a high risk of losing preserved function below the level of injury [65].

A systematic review of the use of the DREZ procedure for neuropathic pain after SCI showed that this treatment may be most effective in patients with specific segmental (dermatomal) pain, as opposed to diffuse pain [66].

Spinal cord stimulators have been used for a variety of chronic pain conditions, including neuropathic pain of various etiologies. The mechanism of action of spinal cord stimulation continues to be incompletely understood. The analgesic effect is postulated to be derived from stimulation of the Aβ fibers within the dorsal column of the spinal cord, which inhibits the afferent transmission of pain information to the brain via the Aδ and C fibers [67].

A systematic review found that spinal cord stimulator is more effective than conventional medical management, and re-operation, in patients with neuropathic pain due to failed back syndrome, and for complex regional pain syndrome type 1 [68].

Furthermore, spinal cord stimulators have also been shown to be effective in the treatment of pain due to diabetic neuropathy. [69, 70]. However, the data on the use of spinal cord stimulation for neuropathic pain after SCI is limited, with one review concluding that there is no significant level of proof to recommend the use of this treatment for this condition [71].

As previously discussed, the use of intrathecal drug delivery may be effective in certain conditions. A recent systematic review found that there is insufficient evidence to recommend the use of intrathecal clonidine, morphine, baclofen, or lidocaine in patients with SCI [72]. However, there is a case study that states that ziconitide may be beneficial for patients with neuropathic pain and spasticity [73].

10. Other Non-Pharmacologic Treatments

Reduction of pharmacologic intervention is important to many patients and practitioners, due to the wide range and high prevalence of adverse effects. Many individuals are concerned about the long-term use of such medications.

As such, there is great interest in the potential benefit that can be derived from physical, non-invasive treatments, and psychological interventions.

A wide variety of such treatments is available, including physical/ occupational therapy, exercise therapy, transcranial electric stimulation (TES), transcranial magnetic stimulation (TMS), transcutaneous electrical nerve stimulation (TENS), acupuncture, osteopathy, cognitive behavioral therapy (CBT), relaxation techniques, and hypnosis.

Recent studies in TES and TMS have demonstrated a modest improvement in post-SCI pain in these patients. These treatments modulate cortical activity by inducing cortical neurons to depolarize, and have been used as an adjunctive treatment in various neurodegenerative disorders such as Parkinson's Disease and Alzheimer's Disease [74]. A systematic review of multiple types of physical treatments stated that TES and TMS may be very promising techniques in providing short and long-term pain relief in patients with neuropathic pain after SCI [75]. This same study also stated that, while generally considered safe for use, treatments such as osteopathy, acupuncture, and TENS have not demonstrated definitive benefit. Additionally, this review showed that psychological therapies such as CBT, hypnosis and visual imagery may be of use in alleviating psychological distress associated with pain. One study examined the effect of exercise on SCI patients, and found a small reduction in the patients treated with exercise, over controls [76]. They also demonstrated gains in physical and psychological well-being. While the authors of this study did not attempt to differentiate between types of pain, these finding suggest that regular exercise can be considered an important component of a comprehensive pain management program for patients with neuropathic pain from SCI.

Conclusion

Neuropathic pain continues to negatively influence the lives of a high percentage of patients with SCI, and is associated with depression, disability, and lost productivity. It is currently a very difficult condition to treat adequately, as many patients continue to live with persistent pain despite attempts at treatment. A multi-disciplinary approach to patient care, in addition to a better understanding of the pathophysiology of neuropathic pain in SCI, will lead to improved diagnosis, management, and treatment of these patients.

Furthermore, research in this area is somewhat limited, with a general lack of well-designed, large, randomized controlled trials.

Hopefully, ongoing research, development of novel medications, and improved management of the acute phase spinal cord injury will lead to more satisfying and reliable treatment options for patients suffering from this condition. By further understanding the pathophysiology through animal models, correctly identifying certain pain subtypes, and using a multidisciplinary team approach, we hope to improve quality of life of patients with SCI-induced central neuropathic pain.

On the basis of our knowledge and experience, we recommend that clinicians first determine the neurologic level of injury and document a complete and detailed history of the patient's pain, including the location, quality, distribution, intensity, periodicity, and duration of the pain, as well as aggravating and alleviating factors.

In the setting of acute pain, it is important to prevent windup or plasticity changes in the central nervous system that may lead to chronic central neuropathic pain. First, we recommend that etiologies such as inappropriate seating positions or equipment, improper transferring techniques, or painful joint positions caused by application of bracing or other assistive devices be corrected. If the pain persists after these corrections, pharmacologic agents may be introduced. In our practice, we use newer antiepileptics, such as pregabalin and gabapentin, or low-dose TCAs such as amitriptyline or nortriptyline as the first line of pharmacologic agents.

If the pain is not sufficiently controlled by one of these agents, we recommend switching to a medication within the same class to see whether one type works better than another. If this still does not relieve the pain, a combination of different classes of medications may be tried. For example, we typically start gabapentin and one of the TCAs. If the patient experiences insufficient relief of pain with this combination, we switch from gabapentin to pregabalin, or from one TCA to another. We reserve opioids as a last resort, used only after various classes of medications or combination therapy fails.

In conjunction with pharmacologic treatment, we recommend a multidisciplinary approach to chronic pain, which includes administration of cognitive behavioral therapy, psychological therapy, regular exercise, sleep optimization, and physical or occupational therapy.

Alternative therapies such as acupuncture, and massage can be used for pain refractory to standard pharmacologic and multidisciplinary approaches. If medications and alternative therapies do not adequately control pain, or if side effects from medications are intolerable, a discussion with the patient regarding invasive interventions such as intrathecal pump, injections, spinal cord stimulator placement, or other surgeries, is warranted.

References

[1] Siddall, P. J., McClelland, J. M., Rutkowski, S. B., Cousins, M. J. A longitudinal study of the prevalence and characteristics of pain in the first 5 years following spinal cord injury. *Pain.* 2003;103(3):249-257.

[2] Murray, R. F., Asghari, A., Egorov, D. D., et al. Impact of spinal cord injury on self-perceived pre- and postmorbid cognitive, emotional and physical functioning. *Spinal cord.* 2007;45(6):429-436.

[3] Stormer, S., Gerner, H. J., Gruninger, W., et al. Chronic pain/ dysaesthesiae in spinal cord injury patients: results of a multicentre study. *Spinal cord.* 1997;35(7):446-455.

[4] Widerstrom-Noga, E. G., Felipe-Cuervo, E., Broton, J. G., Duncan, R. C., Yezierski, R. P. Perceived difficulty in dealing with consequences of spinal cord injury. *Archives of physical medicine and rehabilitation.* 1999;80(5):580-586.

[5] Guirimand, F., Le Bars, D. [Physiology of nociception]. *Annales francaises d'anesthesie et de reanimation.* 1996;15(7):1048-1079.

[6] Bryce, T. N., Biering-Sorensen, F., Finnerup, N. B., et al. International spinal cord injury pain classification: part I. Background and description. March 6-7, 2009. *Spinal cord.* 2012;50(6):413-417.

[7] Treede, R. D., Jensen, T. S., Campbell, J. N., et al. Neuropathic pain: redefinition and a grading system for clinical and research purposes. *Neurology.* 2008;70(18):1630-1635.

[8] Bennett, M. The LANSS Pain Scale: the Leeds assessment of neuropathic symptoms and signs. *Pain.* 2001;92(1-2):147-157.

[9] Ullrich, P. M. Pain following spinal cord injury. *Physical medicine and rehabilitation clinics of North America.* 2007;18(2):217-233, vi.

[10] Bryce, T. N., Richards, J. S., Bombardier, C. H., et al. Screening for neuropathic pain after spinal cord injury with the spinal cord injury pain

instrument (SCIPI): a preliminary validation study. *Spinal cord.* 2014; 52 (5):407-412.

[11] Jensen, M. P. Review of measures of neuropathic pain. *Current pain and headache reports.* 2006;10(3):159-166.

[12] Bouhassira, D., Attal, N., Fermanian, J., et al. Development and validation of the Neuropathic Pain Symptom Inventory. *Pain.* 2004; 108 (3):248-257.

[13] Calmels, P., Mick, G., Perrouin-Verbe, B., Ventura, M. Neuropathic pain in spinal cord injury: identification, classification, evaluation. *Annals of physical and rehabilitation medicine.* 2009;52(2):83-102.

[14] Spinal cord injury facts and figures at a glance. *The journal of spinal cord medicine.* 2013;36(4):394-395.

[15] Oyinbo, C. A. Secondary injury mechanisms in traumatic spinal cord injury: a nugget of this multiply cascade. *Acta neurobiologiae experimentalis.* 2011;71(2):281-299.

[16] Yezierski, R. P. Spinal cord injury pain: spinal and supraspinal mechanisms. *Journal of rehabilitation research and development.* 2009; 46(1):95-107.

[17] Wiesenfeld-Hallin, Z., Aldskogius, H., Grant, G., Hao, J. X., Hokfelt, T., Xu, X. J. Central inhibitory dysfunctions: mechanisms and clinical implications. *The Behavioral and brain sciences.* 1997;20(3):420-425; discussion 435-513.

[18] Gustin, S. M., Wrigley, P. J., Siddall, P. J., Henderson, L. A. Brain anatomy changes associated with persistent neuropathic pain following spinal cord injury. *Cereb. Cortex.* 2010;20(6):1409-1419.

[19] Snedecor, S. J., Sudharshan, L., Cappelleri, J. C., et al. Systematic review and comparison of pharmacologic therapies for neuropathic pain associated with spinal cord injury. *Journal of pain research.* 2013;6:539-547.

[20] Salinas, F. A., Lugo, L. H., Garcia, H. I. Efficacy of early treatment with carbamazepine in prevention of neuropathic pain in patients with spinal cord injury. *American journal of physical medicine and rehabilitation / Association of Academic Physiatrists.* 2012;91(12):1020-1027.

[21] Siddall, P. J., Cousins, M. J., Otte, A., Griesing, T., Chambers, R., Murphy, T. K. Pregabalin in central neuropathic pain associated with spinal cord injury: a placebo-controlled trial. *Neurology.* 2006;67 (10): 1792-1800.

[22] Cardenas, D. D., Nieshoff, E. C., Suda, K., et al. A randomized trial of pregabalin in patients with neuropathic pain due to spinal cord injury. *Neurology.* 2013;80(6):533-539.

[23] Martinez, J. A., Kasamatsu, M., Rosales-Hernandez, A., Hanson, L. R., Frey, W. H., Toth, C. C. Comparison of central versus peripheral delivery of pregabalin in neuropathic pain states. *Molecular pain.* 2012; 8:3.

[24] Finnerup, N. B., Gottrup, H., Jensen, T. S. Anticonvulsants in central pain. *Expert opinion on pharmacotherapy.* 2002;3(10):1411-1420.

[25] Kaptanoglu, E., Solaroglu, I., Surucu, H. S., Akbiyik, F., Beskonakli, E. Blockade of sodium channels by phenytoin protects ultrastructure and attenuates lipid peroxidation in experimental spinal cord injury. *Acta neurochirurgica.* 2005;147(4):405-412; discussion 412.

[26] Hains, B. C., Saab, C. Y., Lo, A. C., Waxman, S. G. Sodium channel blockade with phenytoin protects spinal cord axons, enhances axonal conduction, and improves functional motor recovery after contusion SCI. *Experimental neurology.* 2004;188(2):365-377.

[27] Grunze, H., von Wegerer, J., Greene, R. W., Walden, J. Modulation of calcium and potassium currents by lamotrigine. *Neuropsychobiology.* 1998;38(3):131-138.

[28] Wiffen, P. J., Derry, S., Moore, R. A. Lamotrigine for chronic neuropathic pain and fibromyalgia in adults. *The Cochrane database of systematic reviews.* 2013;12:CD006044.

[29] Finnerup, N. B., Sindrup, S. H., Bach, F. W., Johannesen, I. L., Jensen, T. S. Lamotrigine in spinal cord injury pain: a randomized controlled trial. *Pain.* 2002;96(3):375-383.

[30] Gensel, J. C., Tovar, C. A., Bresnahan, J. C., Beattie, M. S. Topiramate treatment is neuroprotective and reduces oligodendrocyte loss after cervical spinal cord injury. *PloS one.* 2012;7(3):e33519.

[31] Dinoff, B. L., Richards, J. S., Ness, T. J. Use of topiramate for spinal cord injury-related pain. *The journal of spinal cord medicine.* 2003; 26 (4):401-403.

[32] Bray, G. A., Hollander, P., Klein, S., et al. A 6-month randomized, placebo-controlled, dose-ranging trial of topiramate for weight loss in obesity. *Obesity research.* 2003;11(6):722-733.

[33] Song, Z., Meyerson, B. A., Linderoth, B. The interaction between antidepressant drugs and the pain-relieving effect of spinal cord stimulation in a rat model of neuropathy. *Anesthesia and analgesia.* 2011;113(5):1260-1265.

[34] Moulin, D. E., Clark, A. J., Gilron, I., et al. Pharmacological management of chronic neuropathic pain - consensus statement and guidelines from the Canadian Pain Society. *Pain research and management: the journal of the Canadian Pain Society = journal de la societe canadienne pour le traitement de la douleur.* 2007;12(1):13-21.

[35] Sandford, P. R., Lindblom, L. B., Haddox, J. D. Amitriptyline and carbamazepine in the treatment of dysesthetic pain in spinal cord injury. *Archives of physical medicine and rehabilitation.* 1992;73(3):300-301.

[36] Dworkin, R. H., O'Connor, A. B., Audette, J., et al. Recommendations for the pharmacological management of neuropathic pain: an overview and literature update. *Mayo Clinic proceedings.* 2010;85(3 Suppl.):S3-14.

[37] Cardenas, D. D., Warms, C. A., Turner, J. A., Marshall, H., Brooke, M. M., Loeser, J. D. Efficacy of amitriptyline for relief of pain in spinal cord injury: results of a randomized controlled trial. *Pain.* 2002;96 (3): 365-373.

[38] Rintala, D. H., Holmes, S. A., Courtade, D., Fiess, R. N., Tastard, L. V., Loubser, P. G. Comparison of the effectiveness of amitriptyline and gabapentin on chronic neuropathic pain in persons with spinal cord injury. *Archives of physical medicine and rehabilitation.* 2007; 88 (12): 1547-1560.

[39] Kalso, E., Allan, L., Dellemijn, P. L., et al. Recommendations for using opioids in chronic non-cancer pain. *Eur. J. Pain.* 2003;7(5):381-386.

[40] Attal, N., Guirimand, F., Brasseur, L., Gaude, V., Chauvin, M., Bouhassira, D. Effects of IV morphine in central pain: a randomized placebo-controlled study. *Neurology.* 2002;58(4):554-563.

[41] Eide, P. K., Stubhaug, A., Stenehjem, A. E. Central dysesthesia pain after traumatic spinal cord injury is dependent on N-methyl-D-aspartate receptor activation. *Neurosurgery.* 1995;37(6):1080-1087.

[42] McNicol, E. D., Midbari, A., Eisenberg, E. Opioids for neuropathic pain. *The Cochrane database of systematic reviews.* 2013;8:CD006146.

[43] Abs, R., Verhelst, J., Maeyaert, J., et al. Endocrine consequences of long-term intrathecal administration of opioids. *The Journal of clinical endocrinology and metabolism.* 2000;85(6):2215-2222.

[44] Norrbrink, C., Lundeberg, T. Tramadol in neuropathic pain after spinal cord injury: a randomized, double-blind, placebo-controlled trial. *The Clinical journal of pain.* 2009;25(3):177-184.

[45] Sandford, P. R., Benes, P. S. Use of capsaicin in the treatment of radicular pain in spinal cord injury. *The journal of spinal cord medicine.* 2000;23(4):238-243.

[46] Guindon, J., Hohmann, A. G. The endocannabinoid system and pain. *CNS and neurological disorders drug targets.* 2009;8(6):403-421.

[47] Lynch, M. E., Campbell, F. Cannabinoids for treatment of chronic non-cancer pain; a systematic review of randomized trials. *British journal of clinical pharmacology.* 2011;72(5):735-744.

[48] Rintala, D. H., Fiess, R. N., Tan, G., Holmes, S. A., Bruel, B. M. Effect of dronabinol on central neuropathic pain after spinal cord injury: a pilot study. *American journal of physical medicine and rehabilitation / Association of Academic Physiatrists.* 2010;89(10):840-848.

[49] Hagenbach, U., Luz, S., Ghafoor, N., et al. The treatment of spasticity with Delta9-tetrahydrocannabinol in persons with spinal cord injury. *Spinal cord.* 2007;45(8):551-562.

[50] Finnerup, N. B., Biering-Sorensen, F., Johannesen, I. L., et al. Intravenous lidocaine relieves spinal cord injury pain: a randomized controlled trial. *Anesthesiology.* 2005;102(5):1023-1030.

[51] Kvarnstrom, A., Karlsten, R., Quiding, H., Gordh, T. The analgesic effect of intravenous ketamine and lidocaine on pain after spinal cord injury. *Acta anaesthesiologica Scandinavica.* 2004;48(4):498-506.

[52] Herman, R. M., D'Luzansky, S. C., Ippolito, R. Intrathecal baclofen suppresses central pain in patients with spinal lesions. A pilot study. *The Clinical journal of pain.* 1992;8(4):338-345.

[53] Dralle, D., Muller, H., Zierski, J., Klug, N. Intrathecal baclofen for spasticity. *Lancet.* 1985;2(8462):1003.

[54] Jagatsinh, Y. Intrathecal baclofen: Its effect on symptoms and activities of daily living in severe spasticity due to spinal cord injuries: A pilot study. *Indian journal of orthopaedics.* 2009;43(1):46-49.

[55] Kumru, H., Kofler, M., Flores, M. C., et al. Effect of intrathecal baclofen on evoked pain perception: an evoked potentials and quantitative thermal testing study. *Eur. J. Pain.* 2013;17(7):1039-1047.

[56] Taira, T., Ueta, T., Katayama, Y., et al. Rate of complications among the recipients of intrathecal baclofen pump in Japan: a multicenter study. *Neuromodulation: journal of the International Neuromodulation Society.* 2013;16(3):266-272; discussion 272.

[57] Hama, A., Sagen, J. Combination Drug Therapy for Pain following Chronic Spinal Cord Injury. *Pain research and treatment.* 2012;2012: 840486.

[58] Siddall, P. J., Molloy, A. R., Walker, S., Mather, L. E., Rutkowski, S. B., Cousins, M. J. The efficacy of intrathecal morphine and clonidine in the treatment of pain after spinal cord injury. *Anesthesia and analgesia.* 2000;91(6):1493-1498.

[59] Amr, Y. M. Multi-day low dose ketamine infusion as adjuvant to oral gabapentin in spinal cord injury related chronic pain: a prospective, randomized, double blind trial. *Pain physician.* 2010;13(3):245-249.

[60] Gilron, I., Bailey, J. M., Tu, D., Holden, R. R., Weaver, D. F., Houlden, R. L. Morphine, gabapentin, or their combination for neuropathic pain. *The New England journal of medicine.* 2005;352(13):1324-1334.

[61] Chiodo, A. Pain management with interventional spine therapy in patients with spinal cord injury: a case series. *The journal of spinal cord medicine.* 2005;28(4):338-342.

[62] Chun, H. J., Kim, Y. S., Yi, H. J. A modified microsurgical DREZotomy procedure for refractory neuropathic pain. *World neurosurgery.* 2011; 75 (3-4):551-557.

[63] Sindou, M. Surgery in the DREZ for refractory neuropathic pain after spinal cord/cauda equina injury. *World neurosurgery.* 2011;75(3-4):447-448.

[64] Spaic, M., Markovic, N., Tadic, R. Microsurgical DREZotomy for pain of spinal cord and Cauda equina injury origin: clinical characteristics of pain and implications for surgery in a series of 26 patients. *Acta neurochirurgica.* 2002;144(5):453-462.

[65] Sampson, J. H., Cashman, R. E., Nashold, B. S., Jr., Friedman, A. H. Dorsal root entry zone lesions for intractable pain after trauma to the conus medullaris and cauda equina. *Journal of neurosurgery.* 1995;82 (1):28-34.

[66] Mehta, S., Orenczuk, K., McIntyre, A., et al. Neuropathic pain post spinal cord injury part 2: systematic review of dorsal root entry zone procedure. *Topics in spinal cord injury rehabilitation.* 2013;19(1):78-86.

[67] Yampolsky, C., Hem, S., Bendersky, D. Dorsal column stimulator applications. *Surgical neurology international.* 2012;3(Suppl. 4):S275-289.

[68] Simpson, E. L., Duenas, A., Holmes, M. W., Papaioannou, D., Chilcott, J. Spinal cord stimulation for chronic pain of neuropathic or ischaemic origin: systematic review and economic evaluation. *Health Technol. Assess.* 2009;13(17):iii, ix-x, 1-154.

[69] De Vos, C. C., Rajan, V., Steenbergen, W., van der Aa, H. E., Buschman, H. P. Effect and safety of spinal cord stimulation for

treatment of chronic pain caused by diabetic neuropathy. *Journal of diabetes and its complications.* 2009;23(1):40-45.

[70] Daousi, C., Benbow, S. J., MacFarlane, I. A. Electrical spinal cord stimulation in the long-term treatment of chronic painful diabetic neuropathy. *Diabetic medicine: a journal of the British Diabetic Association.* 2005;22(4):393-398.

[71] Lagauche, D., Facione, J., Albert, T., Fattal, C. The chronic neuropathic pain of spinal cord injury: which efficiency of neuropathic stimulation? *Annals of physical and rehabilitation medicine.* 2009;52(2):180-187.

[72] Bensmail, D., Ecoffey, C., Ventura, M., Albert, T. Chronic neuropathic pain in patients with spinal cord injury. What is the efficacy of regional interventions? Sympathetic blocks, nerve blocks and intrathecal drugs. *Annals of physical and rehabilitation medicine.* 2009;52(2):142-148.

[73] Ridgeway, B., Wallace, M., Gerayli, A. Ziconotide for the treatment of severe spasticity after spinal cord injury. *Pain.* 2000;85(1-2):287-289.

[74] Wu, A. D., Fregni, F., Simon, D. K., Deblieck, C., Pascual-Leone, A. Noninvasive brain stimulation for Parkinson's disease and dystonia. *Neurotherapeutics: the journal of the American Society for Experimental NeuroTherapeutics.* 2008;5(2):345-361.

[75] Mehta, S., Orenczuk, K., McIntyre, A., et al. Neuropathic pain post spinal cord injury part 1: systematic review of physical and behavioral treatment. *Topics in spinal cord injury rehabilitation.* 2013;19(1):61-77.

[76] Hicks, A. L., Martin, K. A., Ditor, D. S., et al. Long-term exercise training in persons with spinal cord injury: effects on strength, arm ergometry performance and psychological well-being. *Spinal cord.* 2003;41(1):34-43.

In: Neuropathic Pain
Editor: Alyssa L. Rider

ISBN: 978-1-63321-963-2

Chapter 3

Physiopathology of Neuropathic Pain Following Spinal Cord Injury: New Management Strategies

Pere Boadas-Vaello, Xavier Xifró, Teresa Puig* and Enrique Verdú*

Group of Clinical Anatomy, Embryology,
Neuroscience and Molecular Oncology (NEOMA),
Department of Medical Sciences,
Faculty of Medicine, Universitat de Girona, Girona, Spain

Abstract

Traumatic spinal cord injury (SCI) results in loss of motor, sensory and autonomic functions below the site of injury. About two-thirds of SCI patients develop central neuropathic pain that interferes with daily functioning and ability to participate in life activities, reducing their

* Co-Corresponding authors: Dr. Teresa Puig (teresa.puig@udg.edu) and Dr. Enrique Verdú (enric.verdu@udg.edu). Group of Clinical Anatomy, Embriology, Neurosciencie and Molecular Oncology (NEOMA), Department of Medical Sciences, Faculty of Medicine, Universitat de Girona. C/ Emili Grahit 77, 2ª planta. E-17071 Girona, Spain.

quality of life. Neuropathic pain following SCI is caused by several physio-pathological events that include: (i) disruption of blood vessels associated with hemorrhage, hypoxia, hypoglycemia, and infiltration of neutrophils, monocytes and T-lymphocytes, (ii) necrosis of neurons, glial cells and endothelial cells with the release of potassium ions and glutamate, and (iii) release of cytokines, proteases, prostaglandins and free radicals by infiltrated blood cells and re-activated microglia and astrocytes. All these factors that appeared in the lesion site are able to stimulate nociceptive-specific and wide -dynamic range nociceptive neurons located in the dorsal horn of adjacent spinal cord segments, causing excitation of the anterolateral spinal cord pathway and pain. In addition, these factors also induce central sensitization of nociceptive neurons, and activation of several intracellular signaling pathways that produce genetic and phenotypic changes of nociceptive spinal neurons. These "new" neurons are able to respond more easily to afferent peripheral inputs but also to central pro-inflammatory agents. Then, subjects develop neuropathic pain, including hyperalgesia and allodynia. These types of pain are consuming, chronic and largely refractory to treatment. Thus, new pharmacological treatments or strategies should be developed for reducing neuropathic pain in SCI subjects. The knowledge of the new activated signaling pathways in nociceptive spinal cord neurons after SCI may be crucial for designing novel pharmacological treatments. This chapter gives an overview of the pathological events observed in SCI subjects that develop neuropathic pain, the main intracellular pathways activated in nociceptive neurons during neuropathic pain and new pharmacological approaches focused in phytotherapies such as polyphenols, flavonoids, terpenoids and alkaloids.

Introduction

Spinal cord is a conduit of nerve cells and composed of neurons, glial cells and long interwoven ascending and descending axons that connect various brain and peripheral organs in an organized manner. The spinal cord extends from the base of the brain (medulla oblongata) through the foramen magnum of the skull to the firsts lumbar vertebras (L1 in human or L3 in rats). The spinal cord and its meninges, that from the outside in are the dura mater, arachnoid mater and pia mater, lie within the vertebral canal. The spinal cord is cylindrical, but slightly flattened dorso-ventrally. Histologically, the gray matter of the spinal cord is located centrally, surrounded by white matter. The gray matter is made up of interneurons, the cell bodies and dendrites of efferent neurons, the entering fibers of afferent neurons, and glial cells. The surrounding white matter is composed mostly of groups of myelinated axons, called fiber tracts or spinal cord pathways, run longitudinally through the cord, some descending to relay information from the brain to the periphery, others are ascending to transmit information to the brain. The spinal cord is the part of the central nervous system that controls the voluntary muscles of the limbs and trunk, and which receives sensory information from these regions. It also controls most of the viscera and blood vessels of the thorax, abdomen and pelvis [1, 2].

Spinal cord injury (SCI) results in loss of central control of motor, sensory, and autonomic functions below the site of injury. Most traumatic SCI involve some form of primary blunt mechanical force directed to the spine. Such primary insult may occur following engagement in motor vehicle accidents, collision sports, slips or falls, or violence. Although the spinal cord is relatively protected within the spinal canal, impact to the vertebral column can cause injury to the cord via dislocation or shattering of the vertebrae, disruption of the intervertebral disc or contusion within a stenotic canal [3]. In Spain the incidence of traumatic spinal cord injury was about 24 new cases per million during 2000-2008 [4]. In addition of motor paralysis, sensory anesthesia and autonomic disfunctions, about 62% of patients with SCI showed neuropathic pain [4, 5, 6, 7, 8].

The International Association for the Study of Pain (IASP) defines neuropathic pain as "*pain caused by a lesion or disease of the somatosensory nervous system*". When lesion or disease affects the central somatosensory nervous system, including lesion of spinal cord, thalamus and cortex, this pain is described as central neuropathic pain (IASP Taxonomy). SCI patients showed central neuropathic pain that affects the physiotherapy rehabilitation, the daily activity and their quality of life, causing depression, anxiety and in some cases suicide [9].

The present chapter gives an overview of the clinical and experimental models of SCI and methods for evaluating neuropathic pain, the pathological events observed in experimental and SCI subjects that develop neuropathic pain, the main intracellular pathways activated in nociceptive neurons during neuropathic pain and new pharmacological approaches focused in phytotherapies such as polyphenols, flavonoids, terpenoids and alkaloids.

Clinical and Experimental Models of SCI and Functional Methods for Evaluating Neuropathic Pain

In 1993 Bunge et al., [10] provided a simple classification dividing human SCI into four groups based on gross findings: solid cord injury, contusion-cavity, laceration, and massive compression. Solid cord injury (10% of cases) refers to a cord that grossly appears normal, without evidence of softening, discoloration, or cavity formation, but their damage will be observed by histological examination. Contusion-cavitation injury (49% of cases) shows areas of hemorrhage and necrosis in the cord parenchyma. Laceration (21% of cases) results in clear-cut disruption of the surface anatomy by penetrating missiles or sharp fragments of bone, and their lesions are characterized by a break in the *glia limitans*, with damage to the underlying cord parenchyma. The epicenter of the injury generally shows minimal cavity formation. Finally, in massive compression (20% of cases), the cord is macerated to a varying degree. This lesion is often accompanied by severe vertebral body fractures, and in many instances the epicenter of this lesion is replaced by connective tissue scar [10]. According with these findings, contusion, compression and laceration are the main SCI in human patients.

Using animal models, several experimental procedures have been development to reproduce these human SCI. The first well-documented animal experimentation of SCI was that described by Allen 1991 [11], which used a weight-drop technique on dogs for inducing spinal cord contusion. The technique consists in a dorsal laminectomy on the anesthetized animals for exposing the dorsal surface of the spinal cord. A given weight is dropped from a known height, down a vented guide tube positioned perpendicular to the laminectomy site. As the weight struck the exposed spinal cord, either directly or through an impounder plate that rested on the exposed cord, the underlying tissue is subjected to a dynamic contusion. Depending on the weight and the height, different amounts of force is applied to the cord and resulted in varying degrees of SCI. The weight-drop technique was later adapted for a variety of mammalian species, including monkeys [12, 13], cats [14], sheep [15], rats [16, 17, 18] and mice [19]. After that, several electromagnetic SCI device have been developed including a controlled pneumatic device [20, 21], the New York University (NYU)/MASCIS device [22], the Ohio State University (OSU) device [23, 24, 25] and the computerized Infinite Horizon device [26]. In 2000 Metz et al., [27] compared the spinal cord contusion induced by a weight-drop technique in rats with human chronic SCI. In electrophysiological recordings, prolonged latencies and reduced amplitudes in both motor evoked potentials (MEP) and somatosensory evoked potentials (SSEP) were closely correlated to the impairment of locomotor capacity of lower limbs in rats and humans. The morphological parameters assessed by high-resolution magnetic resonance imaging (MRI) in both species indicated that the lesion length and spinal cord atrophy were significantly related to the electrophysiological and functional outcome parameters. In rats, histological analysis was performed and showed, in addition to the MRI, a close relationship between spared white matter and locomotor capacity. These results suggest an analogous relationship in rats and humans with respect to functional, electrophysiological, and morphological outcomes after spinal cord contusion using the weight-drop technique [27].

Aneurysm clip, calibrated forceps and inflatable extradural balloon catheter are the main experimental techniques for inducing spinal cord injury compression. Aneurysm clip compression consists in a modified Kerr-Lougheed aneurysm clip applying around the exposed spinal cord, with a blade under the ventral surface of the cord and the other over the dorsal surface. The clip, calibrated for a known compression force, is rapidly released and allowed to compress the cord for a predetermined amount of time before release and removal [28]. Other authors have applied compression force-calibrated aneurysm clips vertically and assessed behavior outcome [29]. In both cases, results indicated a high correlation of all neurological outcomes (BBB scale, inclined plane, beam walk) to the compression force. In addition, histological changes, such as the cavity volume, are directly proportional to the force of injury [30, 31, 32]. An alternative to the use of aneurysm clips is a calibrated forceps. A pair of forceps was modified to form an instrument to compress the guinea pig spinal cord laterally, over a 5-mm length, to a thickness of 1.2 mm. This compression injury produced a considerably larger volume of tissue compression. The distribution of damage to axons was similar to that seen following weight-drop contusion trauma in cats. These injuries characteristically resulted in a delayed onset of functional deficits at 1-2 days after injury, followed by a partial recovery over the course of several weeks. Overall, functional outcome correlated significantly with the number of surviving axons in the lesion [33]. In rats, a pair of coverglass forceps with blades 5 mm wide x 0.48 mm thick was used to compress the spinal cord to a thickness from 0.8 to 1.8 mm. Functional outcome does not appear to be a simple linear function of mechanical severity. Rather, functional loss, recovery and tissue damage were constrained to a few discrete levels, especially in mild to moderate injuries. It was demonstrated that the delayed onset of behavioral dysfunction which has been described in the guinea pigsdysfunction, which has been described in the guinea pigs, is absent in the rat, indicating the presence of a significant species difference [34]. Finally, spinal cord compression also was developed using an extradural inflatable balloon. This model uses an inflatable balloon that is introduced in the dorsal subdural space. The spinal cord trauma was graded by varying either the duration of compression or the volume of saline and/or air used to inflate the balloon. Histological results demonstrated that the extent of the spinal lesion was significantly correlated with the physical parameters of compression and with the severity of the behavioral deficit in rats [35]. Complete recovery was seen after 3-5 minutes but not after 7 minutes of 0.1 cc air inflated balloon compression. However, using a 0.2 cc air inflated balloon, no recovery was noted after 1 min compression. These functional results are related with the vascular dysfunctions observed [36, 37].

Of the many traumatic SCI models, the most frequently used methods of injury include complete transection [38, 39, 40, 41], incision, dorsal or lateral hemisection, resection, or aspiration lesions that definitively sever spinal cord axons of passage. Although these types of laceration injuries are not typically seen clinically, they can effectively disconnect both ascending and descending axonal pathways at designated levels of SCI. This approach allows the study of mechanisms that govern the inhibition or successful regeneration of axons across or around laceration injuries as well as of the resulting functional deficits and potential recovery, including pharmacological and cell transplant therapies.

The neuropathic pain following SCI is diagnosed by anamnesis and neurology exploration. The patients are asked about the area of pain, the intensity of pain and they temporal change. The neurology examination includes the exploration of gross pain using cotton and precise pain using von Frey filaments. In some cases also can be used cold and hot objects, the articulation movements and the palpation of soft tissues [42]. In pre-clinical animal models several nociceptive tests have been developed for evaluating neuropathic pain after spinal cord injury, including tail flick test, hot-plate test, plantar test or Hargreave's test, cold plate test, von Frey test and Randall-Selitto test. The tail flick test is one of the oldest nociceptive tests [43]. The measured parameter is the latency (seconds) for tail flick reflex following tail exposure to a heat stimulus that may be applied by dipping the tail tip into a bath at a controlled temperature or by exposing the tail to a controlled infrared heat beam. The hot-plate test [44, 45] is another classic test. The temperature is often set at 52-55ºC, and the measured parameter is the latency for paw licking or the first observed response, which allows repeated measures. Some studies are specifically based on jump latency, particularly in mice. In 1988 Hargreaves et al [46] described a test that differentiates the left and right hind paw responses to heat in freely moving rodents. In this test, animals are placed in clear boxes on a glass surface, and a controlled heat beam system is present below the glass and is moved under a hind paw, and starting the stimulus starts the timer, whereas the paw withdrawal automatically stops the timer. So, the measured parameter is the withdrawal latency to heat stimulus [46]. Cold plates can also be used to assess nociceptive responses after SCI. Rodents are placed into compartment enclosures on the cold surface of the plate, which is maintained at a temperature of 5±0.5ºC. The number of elevations of each hind-paw is recorded for 5 min [47]. All these tests have been designed for evaluating thermal (heat/cold) hyperalgesia, in other words, an increased of pain sensitivity to noxious thermal stimulus.

Mechanical allodynia or pain in response to a non-nociceptive stimulus (e.g. mechanical stimulus) is usually quantified by measuring the hind-paw withdrawal response to von Frey filament stimulation [48]. Rodents are placed into compartment enclosures in a test chamber with a framed metal mesh floor through which the von Frey calibrated monofilaments are applied and thresholds are measured using the up-down paradigm. Finally, the Randall-Selitto test is a classical way to measure mechanical thresholds, mechanical allodynia or hyperalgesia [49]. In this test, the hind-paw is placed between a fixed element, either a surface or a blunt point, and a mobile blunt point exerting a controlled pressure. This pressure is usually provided by a sliding counterweight system. The measured parameter is the threshold (in grams) for appearance of a given behavior, which may be a reflex withdrawal, struggling, or a vocalization, depending on the protocol.

Physiopathology of SCI Related to Neuropathic Pain

Central neuropathic pain is caused by the vascular, biochemical and cellular events that appeared in the injured spinal cord. All these pathological events generate several central agents that stimulate nociceptive neurons located in the dorsal horn of spinal cord segments rostral and caudal to the lesion site. This section focus in explained the main pathological events implicated in the development of neuropathic pain after spinal cord injury (SCI).

Numerous local events within the spinal cord occur immediately after the injury and also contribute to spinal shock. Direct trauma causes necrosis of neurons, endothelial cells, and glia cells. This cell death release glutamate, potassium and cellular enzymes into the extracellular space. These agents diffuse rostro-caudally from lesion site, and potassium causes the activation of microglial cells, whereas glutamate cause the death of nearby neurons and oligodendrocytes through a mechanism called excitotoxicity. Neuron death and oligodendrocytes death with demyelination of ascendent and descendent spinal cord pathways contributes to the sensory, motor and autonomic dysfunctions observed after SCI. However, the diffusion of both agents also causes the hyperexcitability of survived neurons, including nociceptive spinal cord neurons, causing neuropathic pain. Direct trauma also causes breakdown of small blood vessels with the leakage of plasma fluid into the extracellular space. Plasma fluid filled spaces of the spinal cord and contributes to local edema and cell death by mechanical pressure. The diffusion of glutamate and potassium ions also contributes to the cytotoxic edema, occurring mostly in astrocytes. Intracellular swelling of astrocytes alter astroglial functions, including control of molecular transport across the blood-brain barrier (BBB). Other important vascular changes are vasospasm, which is a narrowing of the blood vessels for reducing local edema and hemorrhage. The effects of vasospasm are a decrease of blood flow by 80% and ischemia (e.g. deprivation of neurons and other cells of the oxygen and the other nutrients that they need to survive). The injury of blood vessels also causes hemorrhage with the extravasation of plasma fluid and blood cells mainly erythrocytes. Extravasation of plasma fluid causes an increase of proteases and other plasma proteins in spinal cord parenchyma, such as tissue plasminogen activator (tPA), thrombin, trypsin, and kallikrein-related peptidases. These plasma proteins are able to stimulate glial cells, promote degradation of extracellular matrix components with destabilization of the BBB, and excitation of spinal cord neurons, including nociceptive neurons via plasminogen activator receptors (PARs) [50, 51].

The breakdown of blood vessels also facilitates the infiltration of neutrophils, monocytes and lymphocytes in the injured spinal cord parenchyma. Together to reactive microglia and astrocytes, all these cells facilitate the wound repair of the injured spinal cord. Wound healing is an integration of a coordinated sequence of events involving the release of soluble mediators, extracellular matrix molecules and cellular interactions. The main sequence of events is: inflammation, tissue formation and tissue remodeling. During the inflammation phase the infiltration of blood cells and the reactivation of resident glia cells contributes to the formation of cytokines, chemokines, free reactive radicals, prostaglandins and proteolytic enzymes, soluble mediators that contributes to the degeneration and elimination of cell detritus and facilitates the tissue formation and remodeling, with the formation of a glial scar around the injured spinal cord, demarcating the injured and the penumbra areas [52] The rostro-caudal diffusion of these soluble mediators also promote the excitation of nociceptive neurons and the neurotransmission between the afferent primary nerve fibers and the nociceptive neurons located in the dorsal horn of spinal cord segments surviving to the contusion [53, 54, 55, 56, 57]. The diffusion of prostaglandins (e.g. PGE_2) causes a reduction of the inhibitory glycinergic synaptic transmission in the dorsal horn. Inhibition of glycine receptors occurred via a postsynaptic mechanism involving the activation of EP2 receptors located in nociceptive spinal cord neurons [58]. PGE_2 also induces direct depolarization of nociceptive neurons located in dorsal horn [59]. The diffusion of cytokines and chemokines from lesion site also contributes to the excitation of nociceptive neurons. Interleukin-1β (IL-1β) and tumor necrosis factor alpha (TNF-α) enhance AMPA and NMDA depolarization of nociceptive neurons via TNF-R and IL1R, respectively [57, 60, 61], whereas IL-6 and IL-1β suppressed GABA- and glycine-induced currents in neurons of dorsal horn [60]. CCR2 is constitutively expressed in spinal cord neurons, and their activation by the diffusion of MCP-1 or CCL2 chemokine from lesion site causes a suppression of GABA-induced currents in neurons of dorsal horn [62]. Finally, reactive oxygen species (ROS) that appeared in the lesion site also produce hyperexcitability of wide dynamic range (WDR) neurons [63], and reduce spinal GABA release from inhibitory interneurons located in the dorsal horn [64]. Altogether these findings demonstrated that the diffusion of soluble mediators that appeared in lesion site have able to increase the excitability of nociceptive neurons generating neuropathic pain (Figure 1).

Soluble mediators also contribute to central sensitization of nociceptive neurons and promote long-term potentiation (LTP) of pain synaptic transmission at the dorsal horn (Figure 2). When all of these mediators interact with they receptors located in the nociceptive spinal cord neurons, an influx of calcium and sodium ions were observed. Depolarization of nociceptive neurons and activation of protein-kinases, enzymes implicated in the phosphorylation of NMDA receptors, increased receptor density due to trafficking and enhanced synthesis of ion channels and scaffold proteins [65,

66]. In addition, ROS also modulate the trafficking and phosphorylation of NMDA and AMPA receptors in dorsal horn neurons [67, 68], and TNF-α, IL-1β, and CCL1 also increase NMDA receptor phosphorylation in neurons of dorsal horn [60, 69].

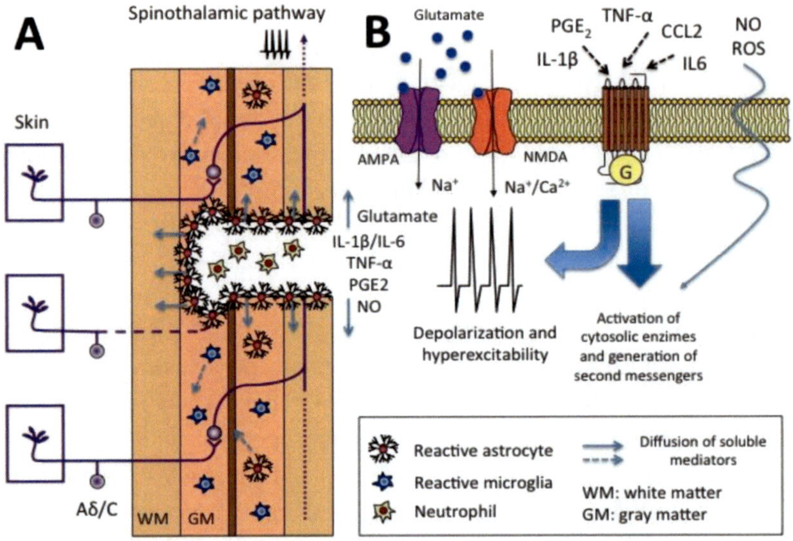

Figure 1. Physiopathology of SCI related with neuropathic pain. [A] Traumatic spinal cord injury causes the re-activation of astrocytes and microglia, and the infiltration of neutrophils and other blood cells. Reactive glia cells generate a glia scar around the injured area. All these cells secrete several soluble mediators (IL-1β, IL6, TNF-α, PGE2, CCL2, NO, ROS) that diffuse by the injured spinal cord parenchyma affecting other glial cells, nociceptive spinal cord neurons, and afferent synaptic terminals of Aδ and/or C nerve fibers (Aδ/C) of nociceptors located in the skin. In the lesion site, the necrotic death of astrocytes and neurons also release glutamate and they diffusion also causes excitation of nociceptive neurons and the propagation of action potentials by the spinothalamic pathway giving neuropathic pain feel. [B] In nociceptive neurons of dorsal horn, these diffusible mediators connect with membrane receptors. Glutamate are able to open ionotropic receptors (AMPA and NMDA) causing an influx of sodium and/or calcium ions (Na^+, Ca^{2+}) that depolarizes nociceptive neurons and generates action potentials that run by spinothalamic pathway. Other mediators interact with metabotropic receptors that modulate ion channels and the excitability of neurons, and that activate several cytosolic enzymes responsible of the generation of several second messengers (cAMP, IP3) that regulate the activity of other enzymes (PKA, PKC, MAPK) and transcriptional factors (NF-kappaB). Finally, other small mediators (ROS, NO) are able to across the cell membrane of nociceptive neurons affecting the excitability and the activity of cytosolic enzymes. For more details see text.

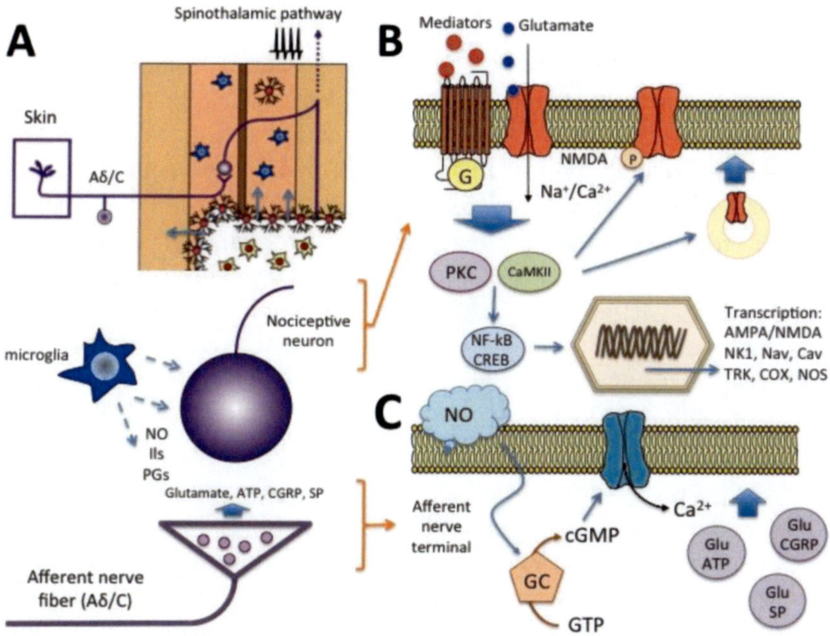

Figure 2. Influence of glutamate and soluble mediators in nociceptive neurons and afferent nerve terminals at dorsal horn. [A] Soluble mediators released by reactive astrocytes and microglia and by neutrophils from the lesion site, together with those secreted by re-active microglial cells near the lesion site, are able to influence the biology of nociceptive neurons and the synapsis between afferent nerve terminals and nociceptive neurons. [B] In nociceptive neurons located in dorsal horn, glutamate and other pro-inflammatory mediators such as interleukins (ILs), nitric oxide (NO), prostaglandins (PGs), are able to facilitate an influx of calcium ions and activation of several enzymes (PKC, CaMKII) responsible of neuronal sensitization by: phosphorylation of NMDA receptor, to increase the trafficking of ionotropic and metabotropic receptors in cell membrane, and to stimulate several transcription factors (NF-kappaB, CREB) that increasing the expression of ion channels, metabotropic receptors, enzymes and other proteins. [C] In afferent nerve terminals, diffusible mediators such as NO facilitates the activation of guanilat cyclase (GC) and the production of cGMP, a second messenger that promote the activation of several ion channels causing influx of calcium ions, that induce the fusion of presynaptic vesicles with presynaptic membrane. The release of neurotransmitters (glutamate, CGRP, SP) from afferent nerve terminals to nociceptive neurons causes hyper-excitability and sensitization of nociceptive neurons at dorsal horn. For more details see text.

Finally, nitric oxide (NO) synthesized by either neuronal or glial cells in the dorsal horn, also contributes to central sensitization and increases neurotransmission between afferent nociceptive fibers and spinal cord nociceptive neurons.

NO acts in afferent nerve fibers facilitating the influx of calcium ions and the delivery of more neurotransmitter (e.g. glutamate, substance-P, CGRP, ATP) over the spinal cord nociceptive neurons and glial cells. When glutamate and substance-P interact with their receptor in nociceptive neurons causes a hyper-excitation of these cells, whereas when glutamate and ATP interact with the glutamatergic and purinergic receptors in microglial cells cause their re-activation, synthesis and secretion of pro-inflammatory cytokines and NO. The interaction of CGRP with pre-synaptic receptors also facilitates pain neurotransmission at the dorsal horn [70]. Similarly, the diffusion of PGE_2 also enhances glutamate release from primary afferent C-fiber terminals via activation of EP1 receptors. The activation of the EP1 receptor initiates an influx of calcium in these fiber terminals that promote the liberation of glutamate and other neurotransmitters over nociceptive spinal cord neurons, including CGRP and ATP [54, 71, 72, 73, 74]. MCP-1/CCL2 chemokine, TNF-α, IL-1β, and ROS enhance the release of glutamate from presynaptic afferent nerve fiber terminals onto nociceptive neurons of substantia gelatinosa and lamina II [75, 76, 77, 78, 79]. All these findings suggest that soluble mediators that appeared in injured spinal cord facilitate long-term potentiation (LTP) of pain synaptic transmission at the dorsal horn of spinal cord segments surviving to the contusion that contributes to the maintenance of neuropathic pain and to the generation of chronic neuropathic pain.

In summary, spinal cord injury causes the generation of several soluble factors such as cytokines (IL1, IL6, TNF-alpha), chemokines (CCL2), prostaglandins (PGE_2), neurotransmitters (glutamate) and ions (potassium) that interacts with nociceptive neurons and afferent primary nerve fibers at the dorsal horn of spinal cord segments rostral and caudal to the lesion site, causing hyper-excitability of spinal cord nociceptive neurons and the pain neurotransmission in the dorsal horn. All of these events induce neuropathic pain in SCI subjects.

Pain Signals Implicated in the Development of Neuropathic Pain

The knowledge of the mechanisms involved in neuropathic pain has attracted considerable interest in the last years to establish efficient pharmacological therapies. As described above, SCI produces anatomical, inflammatory, excitotoxic and neurochemical changes close to the site of injury leading to a change in spinal neuron function. In the spinal cord, pain signals converge onto dorsal horn where nociceptive neurons are located [80]. A large number of studies using different experimental models described that SCI trigger a complex central activation of molecular events. In particular, the release of inflammatory mediators mainly from microglia and activated astrocytes [81], the exacerbated presence of neuromodulators [82] and alterations in ionic channels [83] induces changes in neuronal activity and in long-term synaptic plasticity [84]. This section focus on summarizes these self-continued events in the spinal cord leading to the generation of sustained neuropathic pain.

The Complex Variety of Inflammatory Mediators Following SCI

Inflammatory mediators are the major determinants of neuroinflammation in SCI, and have been shown to contribute to chronic pain. The diffusible inflammatory mediators have been released mainly by both resident and infiltrating immune cells, and may directly sensitize the nociceptive neurons. Glial cells comprise about 70% of the central nervous system and play an important role in maintenance and homeostasis. After SCI, glial cells undergo functional changes with the releasing of inflammatory mediators [85]. Reactive astrocytes and microglia are chronically activated in the spinal cord after clinical [86, 87] and experimental [88] SCI. This pro-inflammatory environment begins at synaptic sites, leading to exacerbate excitation of nociceptive neurons and plastic changes. We next recapitulate the function of some cytokines, chemokines and other inflammatory mediators involved in neuropathic pain following SCI.

Several cytokines have been found to enhance pain, whereas the anti-inflammatory cytokines suppress the effect encoded by pro-inflammatory cytokines. The balance between pro- and anti-inflammatory cytokines is essential to the development of neuropathic pain. In SCI, patients have a systemic increase in levels of pro-inflammatory cytokines, essentially tumor necrosis factor and interleukine-6 and a decrease in levels of anti-inflammatory cytokines. Tumor necrosis factor alpha (TNF-α) is probably the most widely studied pro-inflammatory cytokine. TNF-α acts through two receptors: the constitutively expressed TNFR1 and the inducible TNFR2 [89]. However, although many studies support the role of TNF-α in neuropathic pain, the contribution of its receptors stills controversial. The presence of TNF- α promotes the activation of various signaling pathways related to neuropathic pain, such as the enhanced excitatory postsynaptic currents through glutamate receptors [60] or the activation of nuclear factor-κB (NF-κB), which plays a pivotal role in neuropathic pain [90]. It has been demonstrated using animals models that the interference of TNF-α by neutralizing antibodies or receptor antagonists [91] attenuates neuropathic pain. The TNF-α inhibitor such as infliximab has been tested in peripheral mediated-neuropathic pain models with effective results [92, 93].

In healthy humans, levels of interleukins (IL) are very low, but augment after SCI. It has been showed that the release of IL-1β and 6 in the spinal cord promotes neuropathic pain [91] through increasing glutamate receptors currents, decreasing GABA inhibitory currents and upregulating other inflammatory mediators, such as prostaglandin E2 (PGE_2) or chemokines [60]. The use of inhibitors of IL to reduce their levels in spinal cord attenuates neuropathic pain in different animal models [91, 94]. Some cytokines among them IL-10, IL-4 and tumor growth factor-β (TGF-β), have anti-inflammatory activity. IL-10 can inhibit the release of pro-inflammatory cytokines by the reduction of NF-κB signaling pathway [91]. It has been described that IL-4 decreases the levels of IL-1β and algesic mediators as PGE2 in the spinal cord [95]. Additionally, TGF-β has the capacity to reduce the expression of the chemokine CCL2 [96]. Altogether, the anti-inflammatory cytokines suppress the activation of glial cells, inhibiting the release of pro-inflammatory cytokines, reduced the presence of other inflammatory mediators and also promote the expression of endogenous analgesic mediators.

The magnification of neuropathic pain by cytokines is caused in part by the subsequent activation of other cytokines or inflammatory mediators through the activation of NF-κB pathway. The classical canonical pathway involves several cytokines, such as TNF-α, and also the Toll-like neuronal receptors [97]. The intrathecal administration of antisense oligonucleotides against NF-κB activity attenuates neuropathic pain in a chronic constriction injury animal model [90]. Interestingly, the analgesic effect of nonsteroidal anti-inflammatory drugs (NSAIDs) is related to the inhibition of NF-κB pathway [98]. In the same line, the administration of glucocorticoids reduces hyperalgesia in an animal model of neuropathic pain through the reduction of NF-κB pathway [99].

In the context of neuropathic pain, chemokines enhanced the sensitivity to pain by the attraction of immune cells, activation of microglia and excitation of nociceptive neurons [88]. Two chemokines have been implicated in the generation of neuropathic pain following SCI, the CCL2 (also know MCP-1) and the CX3CL1 (also called fractalkine) [9]. It has been observed that CCL2-mediated signaling is critical for the activation of spinal glia and the developing of neuropathic pain [100]. Interestingly, mice lacking the CCL2 receptor, the CCR2, are resistant to peripheral-mediated neuropathic pain by decreased reactivity of spinal glia and reduced neuronal activation [53]. CX3CL1 is involved in microglial activity and promotes the synthesis of pro-inflammatory cytokines [76]. In the spinal cord, the CX3CR1, the receptor of CX3CL1, is specifically expressed in microglia [101, 102]. CX3CL1 induces nociceptive behaviors by the intracellular phosphorylation of p38 Mitogen-activated protein kinase (MAPK) [103] which], which subsequently stimulates release of pro-inflammatory mediators including Interleukin- 1β, Interleukin-6 or Nitric Oxide [104]. The reduction of the CX3CL1-mediated signaling pathway has an analgesic effect in neuropathic pain models [105]. Additionally, the knockout mice of CX3CR1, the receptor of CX3CL1, showed an important reduction of pain hypersensitivity [106]. Altogether, the studies show an important role of chemokines in the generation of neuropathic pain, resulting interesting targets for the development of analgesic drugs.

A large number of inflammatory mediators are present in the spinal cord following SCI such as bradykinin, histamine and others. However, many works involved in neuropathic pain two receptors-mediated signaling, the purinergic and the PGE_2 receptors. In the spinal cord, the activation of purinergic receptors (P2X) represents a key mechanism involved in neuron-microglia communication promoting the hypersensitivity of nociceptive neurons. In particular, the enhanced activity of P2X results to release of Brain-Derived Neurotrophic Factor (BDNF) [107,108] and this release is critical in the generation of neuropathic pain [109]. BDNF activation of the TrkB receptor down-regulates the expression of the neuronal potassium/chloride co-transporter KCC2 through the Trk B receptor activity [110] contributing a more excitatory environment by the reduction of inhibitory transmission. The inhibition of P2X4/BDNF/KCC2 pathway exerts significant anti-nociceptive effects in neuropathic rats [111].

Prostanoids synthesized through the cyclooxygenase (COX) pathway are known mediators involved in pain. Among them, the PGE_2 have been well studied in different animal models. PGE_2 is derived from the metabolism of arachidonic acid mainly by the action of COX2 and binds to four different receptors, namely EP1 to EP4 [112]. In the spinal cord, EP1 and EP2 seem to be the receptors with nociceptive function. The algesic effect following the intrathecal administration of PGE_2 disappear in EP1 receptor knockout mice [113] and in the presence of EP1 receptor antagonist [74]. The activation of EP1 receptor is related to intracellular calcium mobilizations through the action of phospholipase C/inositol triphosphate, promoting the sensitivity of nociceptive neurons located in the dorsal horn of the spinal cord [112, 114]. The EP2 receptors also contribute to the development of the algesic effect of PGE_2 through the increase of cAMP levels [112] leads to PKA-dependent inhibition of glycinergic transmission [58]. Although poorly data exist about the role of these mechanism in neuropathic pain following SCI, there is evidence that EP1 receptors are up-regulated in the spinal cord of neuropathic pain rats [115,116]. Moreover, it has been reported that inhibitors of COX-2 and the antagonism of EP1 revert the neuropathic pain sciatic ligature-rat model [117]. Taken together, PGE2 shows a role in the maintenance of neuropathic pain. However, more works are needed to determine the therapeutic role of COX-2 inhibitors and EP1 antagonists in neuropathic pain.

The Plasticity of Neuropathic Pain

In the spinal cord, plastic changes that occur following SCI are activated as a recovery mechanism, but it induces several negative consequences as neuropathic pain [118]. These changes are due to the sensitization of the neurons located in the dorsal horn that implies higher synaptic activity, mainly regulated by the presence of the neurotransmitter glutamate [119]. As we mentioned before, the inflammation milieu in the dorsal horn of the spinal cord following SCI induces an increase in the release of glutamate. Moreover, an activation of T-type calcium channels expressed at presynaptic level also contributes to the glutamate release. It has been well described the role of T-channels in peripheral pain, while the localization of these channels in the first lamina of the dorsal horn regulate the release of glutamate and others, such as substance P, to the nociceptive neurons [120]. The increase of intracellular calcium in the peripheral terminals facilitates the release of the neurotransmitters. We next analyze the consequences of the higher release of these neurotransmitters on the nociceptive neurons located in the dorsal horn.

The ionotropic glutamate receptors, AMPA (α-amino-3-hydroxy-5-methyl-4-isoxazolepropionic acid) and NMDA (N-methyl-D-aspartate), mediates the pain signaling due to the excessive release of glutamate in the dorsal horn of the spinal cord. Glutamate presents a higher affinity for NMDA receptors compared to AMPA receptors. However, the presence of the magnesium blocker inhibits the over-activation of NMDA receptors. Thus, glutamate first enhances the activation of AMPA receptor, promoting an increase of intracellular sodium and calcium levels, inducing the deporalization [121]. Then, the continuous activity of AMPA receptor induces a persistent deporalization that leads to the loss of magnesium into the NMDA receptor, facilitating this activity [122] and promoting the hypersensitization of nociceptive neurons. However, is important to note that the metabotropic receptor of glutamate is also involved in the preservation of neuropathic pain following SCI [123].

NMDA receptors are formed by the heteromeric combination of at least one NR1 subunit and one NR2 subunit [124], mainly NR2A or NR2B subunit. The NMDA activity-mediated neuropathic pain is related to the presence of NR2B subunit [125], and not NR2A. It has been described that the NR2A knockout mice not shown pain responses in neuropathic pain models [126]. In contrast, the presence of NR2B facilitates the permeability of calcium through the NMDA receptor. Interestingly, in the spinal cord it has been described that the expression of NR2B is restricted to the dorsal horn [127], and notably in the lamina II [128]. Moreover, the administration of NR2B antagonists produces an analgesic effect through the reduction of the exacerbated synaptic plasticity in the dorsal horn of the spinal cord of neuropathic pain models [129]. Thus, the increase of this subunit is involved in long-term plastic changes that occur in spinal cord [128] that favors the sensitization of nociceptive neurons [130] located in the dorsal horn of the spinal cord.

The activation of the ionotropic NMDA receptor produces the increase of calcium influx resulting in the activation of protein kinases, such as protein kinase C (PKC) [131]. Moreover, activation of other receptors enhances the increase of the PKC-mediated signaling, such as the neurokinin-1 by substance P [93], mediating an over-activation of NMDA receptors [131]. These signal transduction alterations augment the spinal cord synaptic plastic changes and produces the persistent presence of neuropathic pain. These results conduce to the reduction of activation of spinal NMDA receptors by NMDA antagonists to decrease the neuropathic pain related to other causes. In one hand, the use of perzinfotel, a competitive NMDA receptor antagonist, conduces to the reduction of neuropathic pain [132]. In the other hand, noncompetitive NMDA receptor antagonist shows beneficial effects in preclinical and clinical neuropathic pain, such as ketamine [133] or dextromethorphan [134]. However, the long-term use of these compounds is limited by dark effects [93] and more investigations are needed to promote the use of NMDA antagonists in the treatment of neuropathic pain.

The hypersensitivity of the second order neurons of the dorsal horn is not limited to the activation of excitatory neurotransmitters, but also is regulated by the release of inhibitory neurotransmitters by the interneurons [121]. These interneurons have a tonic inhibitory activity through the release of GABA (gamma-amino-butyric-acid) and glycine. In addition, GABA is the principal inhibitory neurotransmitter of the dorsal horn of the spinal cord. In neuropathic conditions, it has been described a reduction of the inhibitory interneurons resulting in over activation of the nociceptive neurons. The inhibition is produced by a reduction of the release of inhibitory neurotransmitters or also by the increase of interneuron death by the exacerbate presence of glutamate [121].

Little information has been given to neuropathic pain spinal mechanisms after SCI compared to the neuropathic pain induced by peripheral injury. However, in the last years, several studies focused their attention in decode the mechanisms involved in neuropathic pain following SCI. Although the cascade does not occur in a known sequential fashion, the mechanisms activated following SCI and conducing to neuropathic pain can be summarized as (i) the presence of inflammatory mediators by the activation of astrocytes and microglia; (ii) the exacerbate sensitivity and activation of the second order neurons placed in the dorsal horn of the spinal cord and (iii) the long-term synaptic changes leading to the activation of spino-thalamic tract.

Phytotherapies As New Pharmacological Treatment of Neuropathic Pain

Several pharmacological treatments have been used for alleviating neuropathic pain in SCI patients, including antiepileptics (valproate, gabapentin, pregabalin, phenytoin), antidepressants (amitryptiline, tramazol), GABA-antagonists (propofol, baclofen), local anesthetics (lidocaine), NMDA-antagonists (ketamine), cannabinoids (dronabinol) and opioids (morphine) [8, 121, 135, 136, 137].

In spite of all these pharmacological treatments, about 50% of SCI patients are refractory and the best pharmacological strategy only reduces the neuropathic pain in about 30% of the SCI patients [6, 8]. The complexity of pathological events implicated in the origin, progress and maintenance of neuropathic pain after spinal cord injury, is one of the possible factors that can to explain these pharmacological effects in SCI patients. In the aim to alleviate central neuropathic pain, new pharmacological strategies will be developed. Phyto-therapy can be a promising strategy for alleviating central and peripheral neuropathic pain. Polyphenols, flavonoids, terpenoids and alkaloids are the main natural products used in experimental animals models of neuropathic pain.

Flavonoids

Flavonoids are diphenylpyrones having two benzene rings linked by a heterocyclic pyrone ring. Several flavonoids have been tested in pre-clinical studies of neuropathic pain, including baicalin, quercetin, pueranin and myricitrin.

Scutellaria baicalensis Georgi is an important medical herb in China for treating the inflammatory diseases and ischemic stroke for thousands of years. A flavonoid compound isolated from S. baicalensis Georgi is Baicalin (BC) which has been proved to posses the anti-oxidant [138], anti-inflammatory [139] and anti-apoptotic properties [140]. After spinal cord contusion BC treatment improve locomotor recovery and spinal cord preservation, and reduce TNF-α, NF-kappaB, caspase-3 and Bax/BcL2 expression [141]. In a rat model of carrageenan-evoked thermal hyperalgesia, BC treatment causes a significant analgesic effect mediated by the inhibition of pro-inflammatory mediator overproduction, including cytokines (TNF-α), nitric oxide, and prostaglandin E2, as well as neurotrophil infiltration [142]. After nerve ligation BC treatment also attenuated the allodynia and hyperalgesia [143].

Quercetin (QUE) is a flavonoid commonly found in food, where it is present in high concentrations in onion, apple, berry, broccoli, caper, tea and wine, and also is an important flavonoid component of a variety of Chinese herbs [144]. QUE scavenges reactive oxygen and nitrogen species [145], targets prominent pro-inflammatory signaling pathways, such as STAT1, NF-κB, and MAPK [146, 147], and phosphodiesterases also to be affected by QUE [148]. QUE attenuates thermal hyperalgesia and cold allodynia in streptozotocin (STZ)-induced diabetic rats [149]. After traumatic spinal cord injury, QUE treatment attenuates the recruitment of neutrophils to the site of injury [150] and promotes the inhibition of the p38MAPK/iNOS signaling pathway mainly in neurons and glial cells [151]. These cellular and molecular spinal changes were related with higher spinal cord preservation and locomotor recovery in QUE-treated animals [150, 151, 152], but changes in nociceptive responses have not reported after SCI.

Puerarin is a major active ingredient extracted from the traditional Chinese medicine Ge-gen (Radix Puerariae, RP), and is one of the three major isoflavonoid compounds of the Kudzu plant (*Pueraria lobata*). After chronic constriction injury, puerarin alleviate neuropathic pain mediated by P2X3 receptors in dorsal root ganglion neurons [153]. On the other hand, it is known that myricitrin, a flavonoid presents in plants of genus Eugenia, comprises anti-nociceptive effects in experimental models of acute and chronic pain [154, 155]. The anti-nociceptive mechanisms of myricitrin include inhibition of PKC, decrease in nitric oxide production, activation of Gi/o protein pathway, alteration of Ca^{2+} and K^{+} movement, and inhibition of p38MAPK phosphorylation in response to cytokines stimulation [154, 156, 157].

Terpenoids

The terpenoids form a large family derived from isoprene units. They are classified depending on the number of isoprene units as hemiterpenes, nonoterpenes, sesquiterpenes, diterpenes, sesterterpenes, triterpenes and tetraterpenes [158]. The tetracyclic triterpene alcohol euphol is the main constituent found in the sap of *Euphorbia tirucalli* [159]. Euphol inhibits mechanical hyperalgesia induced by carrageenan and complete Freund's adjuvant (CFA), and also after peripheral nerve ligation. The mechanisms responsible for euphol analgesic actions are primarily associated with its ability to interfere with the release and/or expression of various inflammatory and pain mediators, such as TNF-α, IL1-β, IL-6, and secondly to interfere with cannabinoid system [160]. Beta-caryophyllene (BCP) is found in large amounts in the essential oils of many common spices and foots plants, such as oregano, cinnamon, clove, rosemary, thyme, and blackpepper [161, 162, 163, 164, 165, 166]. Several health effects have been attributed to BCP or medicinal plants containing BCP including anti-inflammatory [167], local anesthetic [168], anti-carcinogenic [169, 170], anti-fibrotic [171] and anxiolytic activity [172]. In a formalin-induced inflammation and in a partial ligation of sciatic nerve, BCP treatment exerts analgesic effects depending on CB2 signaling [173]. α,β–Amyrin is a pentacyclic triterpene and constitutes the main bioctive component of the resin of *Protium kleinii* and *Protium heptaphyllum* [174, 175]. Moreover, α,β–amyrin exerted a pronounced anti-inflammatory effect in acute models of inflammation [175, 176, 177]. Likewise, this triterpene presented anti-nociceptive supraspinal sites in acute nociception [174]. In addition, α,β–Amyrin decreased IL-1β, TNF-α, IL-6 levels, prevents the activation of NF-κB and CREB, and the expression of COX-2 in spinal cords in inflammatory and neuropathic persistent pain in mice [178].

Alkaloids

Gelsemium elegans Benth is a toxic plant indigenous to Southeast Asia. *G. elegans* extract contains many alkaloids, including gelsenicine, gelsevirine, galsenicine, and koumine [179, 180]. Gelsenicine produced analgesic effect on inflammatory and neuropathic pain in mice [181]. On the other hand, lappaconitine is an alkaloid extracted from the root of the plant Aconitum species. Lappaconitine possesses wide range of biological effects including anti-inflammation [182, 183, 184], antioxidation [184] and anti-nociception [182, 183, 185]. Lappaconitine attenuates the mechanical and thermal hyperalgesia induced by chronic constriction injury, and this analgesic effect involves a decrease of expression and sensitization of P2X3 receptors in DRG neurons [186]. Finally, cassine is a major piperidine alkaloid isolated from the flowers, fruits and leaves of ***Senna spectabilis*** that coexists with espectaline as a mixture of homologous substances [187]. Anti-nociceptive activity of spectaline (a co-metabolite of cassine) has been reported in different models of acute pain, including acetic acid, formalin and capsaicin pain models in mice [188]. Cassine treatment produced a significant inhibition of carrageenan-induced mechanical and thermal nociception in the mouse paw, for reducing the expression of pro-inflammatory cytokines. After CFA injection cassine also reduces the mechanical nociceptive response. The anti-nociceptive effects of this compound seem to be closely associated with its marked inhibition of PGE2 activity, which occurred mainly through blocking the up-regulation of COX-2, MAPK/ERK and NF-κB [189].

Polyphenols

Polyphenols constitute a wide group of different molecular structures that includes catechins, flavones, anthocyanidins, anthraquinones, lignans, coumarins and tannins. Tea is a major source of dietary polyphenols and an even richer source of the flavonols, the catechins and catechin-gallate esters [190, 191, 192]. The epigallocatechin gallate (EGCG) is the most abundant polyphenolic compound in green tea [193, 194]. In experimental models of neuropathic pain such as chronic constriction injury or nerve ligation and after peripheral nerve injury, EGCG treatment causes a reduction of thermal hyperalgesia and mechanical allodynia [195, 196, 197], that is related with a reduction of TLR4, NF-kappaB, TNF-α, IL-1β [196], nNOS and NO [195] expression in the spinal cord. After spinal cord contusion EGCG treatment significantly reduced the expression of TNF-α, IL1-β, iNOS, COX-2, PARP and nitrotyrosine. These biochemical changes are related with higher spinal cord preservation and motor recovery [198, 199]. Intravenous infusion of EGCG following SCI promotes significant locomotor recovery and improves tactile allodynia reflex and mechanical nociception. Paw withdrawal and tail flick latencies increased significantly after EGCG treatment [200]. All these findings suggest that EGCG alleviate peripheral and central neuropathic pain reducing the expression of pro-inflammatory mediators implicated in the excitability of spinal nociceptive neurons, central sensitization and long-term potentation (LTP) of pain synaptic transmission at the dorsal horn.

It is now well established that many polyphenols that include two or more phenolic rings in their chemical structures, such as catechins and flavonoids, act as FASN inhibitors by blocking the ACP, the KR and/or the KS domains in a reversible or irreversible manner [201, 202]. Through a series of thirty-two reactions FASN is able to synthesize long chain fatty acids (LCFA), mainly palmitate (c16), using acetyl-CoA and malonyl-CoA as substrates and NADPH as an electron donor [203], consequently polyphenols reduce palmitate expression in cells. Palmitate is a fatty acid implicated in the S-palmitoylation of proteins. Palmitoylation (or S-palmitoylation) is a posttranslational modification of proteins in which palmitate, or other long-chain fatty acids, is attached via thio-ester linkage to cysteine residues. Hundreds of proteins in eukaryotic cells, including monomeric and heteromeric G proteins, G protein-coupled receptors, ion channels, regulatory enzymes and scaffold proteins are palmitoylated. The addition of palmitate increases the hydrophobicity of a protein and thus may affect their function [204, 205]. It well known that palmitate activates the NF-κB transcription factor and induces the expression of pro-inflammatory cytokines [206, 207, 208]. Palmitoylation also is implicated in the activity and expression of pro-inflammatory enzymes such as iNOS [209, 210, 211] and plays a significant role in controlling channel cell-surface expression and clustering by acting at distinct stages of the trafficking pathway, such as expression and clustering of NR2A and NR2B subunits of NMDA receptors [212]. After SCI, an increase of palmitate expression was reported [213]. All these findings suggest that palmitate and palmitoylation of several proteins such as NF-κB, iNOS and

NMDA receptors can be implicated in the origin and maintenance of neuropathic pain.

In summary, in this section we have exposed experimental evidences that demonstrated the anti-nociceptive role of several natural products including flavonoids, terpenoids, alkaloids and polyphenols affecting neuronal and glial signaling pathways implicated in excitability, central sensitization and long-term potentation of pain synaptic transmission at the dorsal horn of spinal cord.

Acknowledgment

This study was supported by grants from RecerCaixa2010 (Obra Social La Caixa-ACUP), and Accions Singulars de R+D (Sing 12/17) del Vicerrectorat de Recerca de la Universitat de Girona, Spain.

References

[1] Watson C, Kayalioglu G. The organization of the spinal cord. In: Watson C, Paxinos G, Kayalioglu G (eds). *The spinal cord.* 1st edition, Amsterdan, Elsevier, 2009, pp 1-7.

[2] Silva NA, Sousa N, Reis RL, Salgado AJ. From basics to clinical: a comprehensive review on spinal cord injury. *Prog. Neurobiol.* 2014, 114:25-57.

[3] Sekhon LH, Fehlings MG. Epidemiology, demographics, and pathophysiology of acute spinal cord injury. *Spine* 2001, 26: S2-S12.

[4] Pérez K, Novoa AM, Santamariña-Rubio E, Narvaez Y, Arrufat V, Borrell C, Cabeza E, Cirera E, Ferrando J, García-Altés A, Gonzalez-Luque JC, Lizarbe V, Martin-Cantera C, Seguí-Gómez M, Suelves JM. Incidence trends of traumatic spinal cord injury and traumatic brain injury in Spain, 2000-2009. *Accid. Anal Prev* 2012, 46: 37-44.

[5] Siddall PJ, Loeser JD. Pain following spinal cord injury. *Spinal Cord* 2001, 39: 63-73.

[6] Finnerup NB, Jensen TS. Spinal cord injury pain--mechanisms and treatment. *Eur. J. Neurol.* 2004, 11: 73-82.

[7] Cardenas DD, Jensen MP. Treatments for chronic pain in persons with spinal cord injury: A survey study. *J. Spinal Cord Med* 2006, 29: 109-117.

[8] Vranken JH. Neuropathic pain following spinal cord injury. In: Toth C, Moulin DE (eds). *Neuropathic pain: causes, management and understanding.* 1st edition, Cambridge, Cambridge University Press, 2013, pp 145-155.

[9] Cruz-Almeida Y, Felix ER, Martinez-Arizala A, Widerström-Noga EG. Pain symptom profiles in persons with spinal cord injury. *Pain Med* 2009, 10: 1246-1259.

[10] Bunge RP, Puckett WR, Becerra JL, Marcillo A, Quencer RM. Observations on the pathology of human spinal cord injury. A review and classification of 22 new cases with details from a case of chronic cord compression with extensive focal demyelination. *Adv. Neurol.* 1993, 59:75-89.

[11] Allen AR. Surgery of experimental lesion of spinal cord equivalent to crush injury by fracture dislocation of spinal column: A preliminary report. *Journal of the American Medical Association.* 1911, 57: 878–880.

[12] Albin MS, White RJ, Locke GS, Massopust LC Jr, Kretchmer HE. Localized spinal cord hypthermia--anesthetic effects and application to spinal cord injury. *Anesth Analg.* 1967, 46(1):8-16.

[13] Black P, Markowitz RS. Experimental spinal cord injury in monkeys: comparison of steroids and local hypothermia. *Surg Forum.* 1971, 22:409-11.

[14] Faden AI, Jacobs TP, Holaday JW. Thyrotropin-releasing hormone improves neurologic recovery after spinal trauma in cats. *N Engl. J. Med.* 1981, Oct 29;305(18): 1063-7.

[15] Yeo JD, Payne W, Hinwood B, Kidman AD. The experimental contusion injury of the spinal cord in sheep. Paraplegia. 1975, 12(4): 279-98.

[16] Noble LJ, Wrathall JR. Spinal cord contusion in the rat: morphometric analyses of alterations in the spinal cord. *Exp. Neurol.* 1985, Apr;88(1):135-49.

[17] Panjabi MM1, Wrathall JR. Biomechanical analysis of experimental spinal cord injury and functional loss. *Spine* (Phila Pa 1976). 1988, 13(12): 1365-70.

[18] Wrathall JR, Pettegrew RK, Harvey F. Spinal cord contusion in the rat: production of graded, reproducible, injury groups. *Exp. Neurol.* 1985, 88(1): 108-22.

[19] Kuhn PL, Wrathall JR. A mouse model of graded contusive spinal cord injury. *J. Neurotrauma.* 1998, 15(2): 125-40.

[20] Anderson TE. A controlled pneumatic technique for experimental spinal cord contusion. *J. Neurosci Methods.* 1982, 6(4): 327-33.

[21] Kearney PA, Ridella SA, Viano DC, Anderson TE. Interaction of contact velocity and cord compression in determining the severity of spinal cord injury. *J. Neurotrauma.* 1988, 5(3): 187-208.

[22] Gruner JA. A monitored contusion model of spinal cord injury in the rat. *J. Neurotrauma.* 1992, 9(2): 123-8.

[23] Noyes DH. Correlation between parameters of spinal cord impact and resultant injury. *Exp. Neurol.* 1987, 95(3): 535-47.

[24] Noyes DH. Electromechanical impactor for producing experimental spinal cord injury in animals. *Med. Biol. Eng. Comput.* 1987, 25(3): 335-40.

[25] Bresnahan JC, Beattie MS, Todd FD 3rd, Noyes DH. A behavioral and anatomical analysis of spinal cord injury produced by a feedback-controlled impaction device. *Exp. Neurol.* 1987, 95(3): 548-70.

[26] Scheff SW, Rabchevsky AG, Fugaccia I, Main JA, Lumpp JE Jr. Experimental modeling of spinal cord injury: characterization of a force-defined injury device. *J. Neurotrauma.* 2003, 20(2): 179-93.

[27] Metz GA, Curt A, van de Meent H, Klusman I, Schwab ME, Dietz V. Validation of the weight-drop contusion model in rats: a comparative study of human spinal cord injury. *J. Neurotrauma.* 2000, 17(1): 1-17.

[28] Rivlin AS, Tator CH. Effect of duration of acute spinal cord compression in a new acute cord injury model in the rat. Surg Neurol. 1978, 10(1): 38-43.

[29] von Euler M, Seiger A, Sundström E. Clip compression injury in the spinal cord: a correlative study of neurological and morphological alterations. *Exp. Neurol.* 1997, 145(2 Pt 1): 502-10.

[30] Fehlings MG, Tator CH. The relationships among the severity of spinal cord injury, residual neurological function, axon counts, and counts of retrogradely labeled neurons after experimental spinal cord injury. *Exp. Neurol.* 1995, 132(2): 220-8.

[31] Poon PC, Gupta D, Shoichet MS, Tator CH. Clip compression model is useful for thoracic spinal cord injuries: histologic and functional correlates. *Spine* (Phila Pa 1976). 2007, 1;32(25): 2853-9.

[32] Plemel JR, Duncan G, Chen KW, Shannon C, Park S, Sparling JS, Tetzlaff W. A graded forceps crush spinal cord injury model in mice. *J. Neurotrauma*. 2008, 25(4): 350-70.

[33] Blight AR. Morphometric analysis of a model of spinal cord injury in guinea pigs, with behavioral evidence of delayed secondary pathology. *J. Neurol. Sci.* 1991, 103(2): 156-71.

[34] Gruner JA1, Yee AK, Blight AR. Histological and functional evaluation of experimental spinal cord injury: evidence of a stepwise response to graded compression. *Brain Res*. 1996, 5;729(1):90-101.

[35] Martin D1, Schoenen J, Delrée P, Gilson V, Rogister B, Leprince P, Stevenaert A, Moonen G. Experimental acute traumatic injury of the adult rat spinal cord by a subdural inflatable balloon: methodology, behavioral analysis, and histopathology. *J. Neurosci. Res*. 1992, 32(4): 539-50.

[36] Khan M, Griebel R. Acute spinal cord injury in the rat: comparison of three experimental techniques. *Can. J. Neurol. Sci*. 1983, 10(3):161-5.

[37] Khan M, Griebel R, Rozdilsky B, Politis M. Hemorrhagic changes in experimental spinal cord injury models. *Can. J. Neurol. Sci*. 1985, 12(3): 259-62.

[38] Feringa ER, Kinning WK, Britten AG, Vahlsing HL. Recovery in rats after spinal cord injury. *Neurology*. 1976, 26(9): 839-43.

[39] Feringa ER, Vahlsing HL, Smith BE. Retrograde transport in corticospinal neurons after spinal cord transection. *Neurology*. 1983, 33(4): 478-82.

[40] Feringa ER, Lee GW, Vahlsing HL, Gilbertie WJ. Cell death in the adult rat dorsal root ganglion after hind limb amputation, spinal cord transection, or both operations. *Exp. Neurol*. 1985, 87(2): 349-57.

[41] Fehlings MG, Tator CH, Linden RD, Piper IR. Motor evoked potentials recorded from normal and spinal cord-injured rats. *Neurosurgery*. 1987, 20(1): 125-30.

[42] Werhagen L1, Budh CN, Hultling C, Molander C. Neuropathic pain after traumatic spinal cord injury--relations to gender, spinal level, completeness, and age at the time of injury. *Spinal Cord*. 2004, 42(12): 665-73.

[43] Fred E. D'amour, Donn L. Smith. A method for determining loss of pain sensation. *J. Pharmacol Exp Ther*. 1941, 72:74-79.

[44] G. Woolfe, A. D. Macdonald. The evaluation of the analgesic action of pethidine hydrochloride (Demerol). *J. Pharmacol. Exp. Ther*. 1944, 80(3): 300-307.

[45] O'Callaghan, J.P., Holtzman, S.G. Quantification of the analgesic activity of narcotic antagonists by a modified hot-plate procedure. *J. Pharmacol. Exp. Therapeut.* 1975, 192(3): 1.

[46] Hargreaves K, Dubner R, Brown F, Flores C, Joris J. A new and sensitive method for measuring thermal nociception in cutaneous hyperalgesia. *Pain.* 1988, 32(1): 77-88.

[47] Bennett GJ, Xie YK. A peripheral mononeuropathy in rat that produces disorders of pain sensation like those seen in man. *Pain.* 1988, 33(1):87-107.

[48] Chaplan SR, Bach FW, Pogrel JW, Chung JM, Yaksh TL. Quantitative assessment of tactile allodynia in the rat paw. *J. Neurosci Methods.* 1994, 53(1): 55-63.

[49] Randall L.O. Selitto J.J. A method for measurement of analgesic activity on inflammed tissue. *Arch. Int. Pharmacodyn. Ther.* 1957, ;111: 409–419.

[50] Narita M, Usui A, Narita M, Niikura K, Nozaki H, Khotib J, Nagumo Y, Yajima Y, Suzuki T. Protease-activated receptor-1 and platelet-derived growth factor in spinal cord neurons are implicated in neuropathic pain after nerve injury. *J. Neurosci.* 2005, 25(43): 10000-9.

[51] Gieseler F, Ungefroren H, Settmacher U, Hollenberg MD, Kaufmann R. Proteinase-activated receptors (PARs) - focus on receptor-receptor-interactions and their physiological and pathophysiological impact. *Cell Commun Signal.* 2013, 11:86.

[52] Bethea JR. Spinal cord injury-induced inflammation: a dual-edged sword. *Prog. Brain Res.* 2000, 128:33-42.

[53] Abbadie C, Bhangoo S, De Koninck Y, Malcangio M, Melik-Parsadaniantz S, White FA. Chemokines and pain mechanisms. *Brain Res Rev.* 2009, 60(1): 125-34.

[54] Miller RJ, Jung H, Bhangoo SK, White FA. Cytokine and chemokine regulation of sensory neuron function. *Handb Exp Pharmacol.* 2009, (194): 417-49.

[55] White FA, Feldman P, Miller RJ. Chemokine signaling and the management of neuropathic pain. *Mol Interv.* 2009, 9(4): 188-95.

[56] Spicarova D, Nerandzic V, Palecek J. Modulation of spinal cord synaptic activity by tumor necrosis factor α in a model of peripheral neuropathy. *J. Neuroinflammation.* 2011, 8:177.

[57] Liu T, Jiang CY, Fujita T, Luo SW, Kumamoto E. Enhancement by interleukin-1β of AMPA and NMDA receptor-mediated currents in adult rat spinal superficial dorsal horn neurons. *Mol Pain.* 2013, 28;9:16.

[58] Ahmadi S, Lippross S, Neuhuber WL, Zeilhofer HU. PGE(2) selectively blocks inhibitory glycinergic neurotransmission onto rat superficial dorsal horn neurons. *Nat Neurosci.* 2002, 5(1): 34-40.

[59] Baba, H., Kohno, T., Moore, K.A., Woolf, C.J. Direct activation of rat spinal dorsal horn neurons by prostaglandin E2. *J. Neurosci.* 2001, 21(5): 1750-6.

[60] Kawasaki Y, Zhang L, Cheng JK, Ji RR. Cytokine mechanisms of central sensitization: distinct and overlapping role of interleukin-1beta, interleukin-6, and tumor necrosis factor-alpha in regulating synaptic and neuronal activity in the superficial spinal cord. *J. Neurosci.* 2008, 28(20): 5189-94.

[61] Zhang L, Berta T, Xu ZZ, Liu T, Park JY, Ji RR. TNF-α contributes to spinal cord synaptic plasticity and inflammatory pain: distinct role of TNF receptor subtypes 1 and 2. *Pain.* 2011, 152(2): 419-27.

[62] Gosselin RD1, Varela C, Banisadr G, Mechighel P, Rostene W, Kitabgi P, Melik-Parsadaniantz S. Constitutive expression of CCR2 chemokine receptor and inhibition by MCP-1/CCL2 of GABA-induced currents in spinal cord neurones. *J. Neurochem.* 2005, 95(4): 1023-34.

[63] Y. Gwak, C. Hulsebosch. Reactive oxygen species (ROS) mediated neuropathic pain signaling following spinal cord injury. *The Journal of Pain* 2012, 13 (4): S56.

[64] Yowtak J, Lee KY, Kim HY, Wang J, Kim HK, Chung K, Chung JM. Reactive oxygen species contribute to neuropathic pain by reducing spinal GABA release. *Pain.* 2011, 152(4): 844-52.

[65] Costigan M, Scholz J, Woolf CJ. Neuropathic pain: a maladaptive response of the nervous system to damage. *Annu Rev Neurosci.* 2009, 32:1-32.

[66] Latremoliere A, Woolf CJ. Central sensitization: a generator of pain hypersensitivity by central neural plasticity. *J. Pain.* 2009, 10(9): 895-926.

[67] Gao X, Kim HK, Chung JM, Chung K. Reactive oxygen species (ROS) are involved in enhancement of NMDA-receptor phosphorylation in animal models of pain. *Pain.* 2007, 131(3): 262-71.

[68] Lee DZ, Chung JM, Chung K, Kang MG. Reactive oxygen species (ROS) modulate AMPA receptor phosphorylation and cell-surface localization in concert with pain-related behavior. *Pain.* 2012, 153(9): 1905-15.

[69] Akimoto N, Honda K, Uta D, Beppu K, Ushijima Y, Matsuzaki Y, Nakashima S, Kido MA, Imoto K, Takano Y, Noda M. CCL-1 in the

spinal cord contributes to neuropathic pain induced by nerve injury. *Cell Death Dis.* 2013, 20;4: e679.

[70] Rygh LJ, Tjølsen A, Hole K, Svendsen F. Cellular memory in spinal nociceptive circuitry. *Scand J Psychol.* 2002, 43(2): 153-9.

[71] Ferreira SH, Lorenzetti BB. Intrathecal administration of prostaglandin E2 causes sensitization of the primary afferent neuron via the spinal release of glutamate. *Inflamm Res.* 1996, 45(10): 499-502.

[72] Malmberg AB, Yaksh TL. The effect of morphine on formalin-evoked behaviour and spinal release of excitatory amino acids and prostaglandin E2 using microdialysis in conscious rats. *Br. J. Pharmacol.* 1995, 114(5): 1069-75.

[73] R.A. Coleman, W.L. Smith, S. Narumiya. International union of pharmacology classification of prostanoid receptors: properties, distribution, and structure of the receptors and their subtypes, *Pharmacol. Rev.* 1994, 46:205–229.

[74] Nakayama Y, Omote K, Kawamata T, Namiki A. Role of prostaglandin receptor subtype EP1 in prostaglandin E2-induced nociceptive transmission in the rat spinal dorsal horn. *Brain Res.* 2004, 1010(1-2): 62-8.

[75] Gustafson-Vickers SL, Lu VB, Lai AY, Todd KG, Ballanyi K, Smith PA. Long-term actions of interleukin-1beta on delay and tonic firing neurons in rat superficial dorsal horn and their relevance to central sensitization. *Mol Pain.* 2008, 4:63.

[76] Gao YJ, Zhang L, Samad OA, Suter MR, Yasuhiko K, Xu ZZ, Park JY, Lind AL, Ma Q, Ji RR. JNK-induced MCP-1 production in spinal cord astrocytes contributes to central sensitization and neuropathic pain. *J. Neurosci.* 2009, 29(13): 4096-108.

[77] Gruber-Schoffnegger D, Drdla-Schutting R, Hönigsperger C, Wunderbaldinger G, Gassner M, Sandkühler J. Induction of thermal hyperalgesia and synaptic long-term potentiation in the spinal cord lamina I by TNF-α and IL-1β is mediated by glial cells. *J. Neurosci.* 2013, 33(15): 6540-51.

[78] Nishio N, Taniguchi W, Sugimura YK, Takiguchi N, Yamanaka M, Kiyoyuki Y, Yamada H, Miyazaki N, Yoshida M, Nakatsuka T. Reactive oxygen species enhance excitatory synaptic transmission in rat spinal dorsal horn neurons by activating TRPA1 and TRPV1 channels. *Neuroscience.* 2013, 247:201-12.

[79] Yan X, Weng HR. Endogenous interleukin-1β in neuropathic rats enhances glutamate release from the primary afferents in the spinal

dorsal horn through coupling with presynaptic N-methyl-D-aspartic acid receptors. *J. Biol. Chem.* 2013, 288(42): 30544-57.

[80] Gerbhardt, G.F. Descending modulation of pain. *Neurosci. Biobehav. Rev.* 2004, 27:729-737.

[81] Watkins, L.R., Maiser, S.F. Glia: a novel drug discovery target for clinical pain. *Nat. Rev. Drug Discov.* 2003, 2:973-985 .

[82] D'Angelo, R., Morreale, A., Donadio, V., Boriani, S., Maraldi, N., Plazzi, G., Liguori, R. Neuropathic pain following spinal cord injury: what we know about mechanisms, assessment and management. *Eur. Rev. Med. Parmacol. Sci.* 2013, 17: 3257-3261.

[83] Hans, B.C., Waxman, S.G. Sodium channel expression and the molecular pathophysiology of pain after SCI. *Prog. Brain Res.* 2007, 161: 195-203.

[84] Ji, R.R., Woolf, C.J. Neuronal plasticity and signal transduction in nociceptive neurons: implication for the initiations and mateinance of pathological pain. *Neurobiol. Dis.* 2001, 8: 1-10.

[85] Mika, J., Zychowska, M., Popiolek-Barczyk, K., Rojewska, E., Przewlocka, B. Importance of glial activation in neuropathic pain. *Eur. J. Pharmacol.* 2013, 716: 106-119.

[86] Schmitt, A.B., Buss, A., Breuer, S., Brook, G.A., Pech, K., Martin, D., Schoenen, J., Noth, J., Love, S., Schröder, J.M., Kreutzberg, G.W., Nacimiento, W. Major histocompatibility complex class II expression by activated microglia caudal to lesions of descending tracts in the human spinal cord is not associated with a T cell response. *Acta Neuropathol.* 2000, 100: 528-536.

[87] Chang, H.T. Subacute human spinal cord contusion: few lymphocytes and many macrophages. *Spinal Cord* 2006, 45: 174-182.

[88] Hulsebosch, C.E., Hains, B.C., Crown, E.D., Carlton, S.M. Mechanisms of chronic central neuropathic pain after spinal cord injury. *Brain Res.* Rev. 2009, 60: 202-213.

[89] Locksley, R.M., Killeen, N., Lenardo, M.J. The TNF and TNF receptor superfamilies: integrating mammalian biology. *Cell.* 2001, 104: 487-501.

[90] Sun, T., Song, W.G., Fu, Z.J., Liu, Z.H., Liu, Y.M., Yao, S.L. Alleviation of neuropathic pain by intrathecal injection of antisense oligonucleotides to p65 subunit of NF-kappaB. *Br. J. Anaesth.* 2006, 97: 553-558.

[91] Austin, P.J., Moalem-Taylor, G. The neuro-immune balance in neuropathic pain: involvement of inflammatory immune cells, immune-like glial cells and cytokines. *J. Neuroimmunol.* 2010, 229: 26-50.

[92] Sommer, C., Schafers, M., Marziniak, M., Toyka, K.V. Ertanecept reduces hyperalgesia in experimental painful neuropathy. *J. Peripher. Nerv. Syst.* 2001, 6: 67-72.

[93] Cohen, S.P., Mao, J. Neuropathic pain: mechanisms and their clinical implications. *BMJ* 2014, 348: f7656.

[94] Dominguez, E., Mauborgne, A., Mallet, J., Desclaux, M., Pohl, M. SOCS3-mediated blockade of JAK/STAT3 signaling pathway reveals its major contribution to spinal cord neuroinflammation and mechanical allodynia after peripheral nerve injury. *J. Neurosci.* 2010, 30: 5754-5766.

[95] Hao, S., Mata, M., Glorioso, J.C., Fink, D.J. HSV-mediated expression of interleukin-4 in dorsal root ganglion neurons reduces neuropathic pain. *Mol. Pain* 2006, 2:6.

[96] Echeverry, S., Shi, X.Q., Haw, A., Liu, H., Zhang, Z.W., Zhang, J. Transforming growth factor-beta1 impairs neuropathic pain through pleiotropic effect. *Mol. Pain* 2009, 5:16.

[97] Niederberger, E., Geisslinger, G. The IKK-NF-κB pathway: a source for novel molecular drug targets in pain therapy? *FASEB J.* 2008, 22: 3432-3442.

[98] Yin, M.J., Yamamoto, Y., Gaynor, R.B. The anti-inflammatory agents aspirin and salicylate inhibit the activity of I(kappa)B kinase-beta. *Nature.* 1998, 396:77-80.

[99] Xie, W., Liu, X., Xuan, H., Luo, S., Zhao, X., Zhou, Z., Xu, J. Effect of betamethasone on neuropathic pain and cerebral expression of NF-kappaB and cytokines. *Neurosci. Lett.* 2006, 393: 255-259.

[100] Thacker, M.A., Clark, A.K., Bishop, T., Grist, J., Yip, P.K., Moon, L.D., Thompson, S.W., Marchand, F., McMahon, S.B. CCL2 is a key mediator of microglia activation in neuropathic pain states. *Eur. J. Pain* 2009, 13: 263-272.

[101] Lindia, J. A., McGowan, E., Jochnowitz, N., Abbadie, C. Induction of CX3CL1 expression in astrocytes and CX3CR1 in microglia in the spinal cord of a rat model of neuropathic pain. *J. Pain* 2005, 6: 434–438.

[102] Verge, G. M., Milligan, E. D., Maier, S. F., Watkins, L. R., Naeve, G. S., Foster, A. C. Fractalkine (CX3CL1) and fractalkine receptor (CX3CR1) distribution in spinal cord and dorsal root ganglia under basal and neuropathic pain conditions. *Eur. J. Neurosci.* 2004, 20: 1150-1160.

[103] Zhuang, Z. Y., Kawasaki, Y., Tan, P. H., Wen, Y. R., Huang, J., Ji, R. R. Role of the CX3CR1/p38 MAPK pathway in spinal microglia for the development of neuropathic pain following nerve injury-induced cleavage of fractalkine. *Brain Behav. Immun.* 2007, 21: 642–651

[104] Milligan, E.D., Zapata, V., Schoeniger, D., Chacur, M., Green, P., Poole, S. An initial investigation of spinal mechanisms underlying pain enhancement induced by fractalkine, a neuronally released chemokine. *Eur. J. Neurosci.* 2005, 22: 2775–2782.

[105] Milligan, E.D., Zapata, V., Chacur, M., Schoeniger, D., Biedenkapp, J., O'Connor, K.A., Verge, G.M., Chapman, G., Green, P., Foster, A.C., Naeve, G.S., Maier, S.F., Watkins, L.R. Evidence that exogenous and endogenous fractalkine can induce spinal nociceptive facilitation in rats. *Eur. J. Neurosci.* 2004, 20: 2294-2302

[106] Staniland, A.A., Clark, A.K., Wodarski, R., Sasso, O., Maione, F., D'Acquisto, F., Malcangio, M. Reduced inflammatory and neuropathic pain and decreased spinal microglial response in fractalkine receptor (CX3CR1) knockout mice. *J. Neurochem.* 2010, 114: 1143-1157.

[107] Ulmann, L., Hatcher, J. P., Hughes, J. P., Chaumont, S., Green, P. J., Conquet, F. Up-regulation of P2X4 receptors in spinal microglia after peripheral nerve injury mediates BDNF release and neuropathic pain. *J. Neurosci.* 2008, 28: 11263–11268.

[108] Trang, T., Beggs, S., Wan, X., Salter, M. W. P2X4-receptor-mediated synthesis and release of brain-derived neurotrophic factor in microglia is dependent on calcium and p38-mitogen-activated protein kinase activation. *J. Neurosci.* 2009, 29: 3518–3528.

[109] Tsuda, M., Shigemoto-Mogami, Y., Koizumi, S., Mizokoshi, A., Kohsaka, S., Salter, M. W. P2X4 receptors induced in spinal microglia gate tactile allodynia after nerve injury. *Nature* 2003, 424: 778–783.

[110] Coull, J. A., Beggs, S., Boudreau, D., Boivin, D., Tsuda, M., Inoue, K. BDNF from microglia causes the shift in neuronal anion gradient underlying neuropathic pain. *Nature* 2005, 438: 1017–1021.

[111] Gagnon, M., Bergeron, M. J., Lavertu, G., Castonguay, A., Tripathy, S., Bonin, R. P. Chloride extrusion enhancers as novel therapeutics for neurological diseases. *Nat. Med.* 2013, 19: 1524–1528.

[112] Breyer, R.M., Bagdassarian, C.K., Myers, S.A., Breyer, M.D. Prostanoid receptors: subtypes and signaling. *Annu. Rev. Pharmacol. Toxicol.* 2001, 41:661-690.

[113] Minami, T., Nakano, H., Kobayashi, T., Sugimoto, Y., Ushikubi, F., Ichikawa, A., Narumiya, S., Ito, S. Characterization of EP receptor

subtypes responsible for prostaglandin E2-induced pain responses by use of EP1 and EP3 receptor knockout mice. 2001, *Br. J. Pharmacol.* 2001, 133: 438-444.

[114] Hall A, Brown SH, Budd C, Clayton NM, Giblin GM, Goldsmith P, Hayhow TG, Hurst DN, Naylor A, Anthony Rawlings D, Scoccitti T, Wilson AW, Winchester WJ. Discovery of GSK345931A: An EP(1) receptor antagonist with efficacy in preclinical models of inflammatory pain. *Bioorg. Med. Chem. Lett.* 2009, 19: 497-501.

[115] Ma, W., Eisenach, J.C. Four PGE2 EP receptors are up-regulated in injured nerve following partial sciatic nerve ligation. *Exp. Neurol.* 2003, 183: 581-592.

[116] Woodhams, P.L., MacDonald, R.E., Collins, S.D., Chessell, I.P., Day, N.C. Localisation and modulation of prostanoid receptors EP1 and EP4 in the rat chronic constriction injury model of neuropathic pain. *Eur. J. Pain.* 2007, 11: 605-613.

[117] Kawahara, H., Sakamoto, A., Takeda, S., Onodera, H., Imaki, J., Ogawa, R. A. prostaglandin E2 receptor subtype EP1 receptor antagonist (ONO-8711) reduces hyperalgesia, allodynia, and c-fos gene expression in rats with chronic nerve constriction. *Anesth. Analg.* 2001, 93: 1012-1017.

[118] Brown, A., Weaver, L.C. The dark side of neuroplasticity. *Exp. Neurol.* 2012, 235: 133-141.

[119] Woolf, C.J. Central sensitization: implications for the diagnosis and treatment of pain. *Pain.* 2011, 152: S2-S15.

[120] Zamponi, G.W., Lewis, R.J., Todorovic, S.M., Arneric, S.P. Snutch, T.P. Role of voltage-gated calcium channels in ascending pain pathways. *Brain Res.* 2009, 60: 84-89.

[121] Vranken, J.H. Elucidation of pathophysiology and treatment of neuropathic pain. *Cent. Nerv. Syst. Agents Med. Chem.* 2009, 9: 71-78.

[122] Larsson, M., Broman, J., Synaptic plasticity and pain: role of ionotropic glutamate receptors. *Neuroscientist.* 2011, 17: 256-273.

[123] Mills, C.D., Johnson, K.M., Hulsebosch, C.E. Group I metabotropic glutamate receptors in spinal cord injury: roles in neuroprotection and the development of chronic central pain. *J. Neurotrauma.* 2002, 19: 23-42.

[124] Cull-Candy, S., Brickley, S., Farrant, M. NMDA receptor subunits: diversity, development and disease. *Curr. Opin. Neurobiol.* 2001, 11: 327–335.

[125] Wu, L.J., Zhuo, M. Targeting the NMDA receptor subunit NR2B for the treatment of neuropathic pain. *Neurotherapeutics.* 2009, 6: 693-702.

[126] Petrenko, A.B., Yamakura, T., Baba, H., Sakimura, K. Unaltered pain-related behavior in mice lacking NMDA receptor GluRepsilon 1 subunitUnaltered painrelated behavior in mice lacking NMDA receptor GluR_ 1 subunit. *Neurosci. Res.* 2003, 46: 199 –204.

[127] Watanabe, M., Inoue, Y., Sakimura, K., Mishina, M. Developmental changes in distribution of NMDA receptor channel subunit mRNAs. *Neuroreport.* 1992, 3: 1138–1140.

[128] Boyce, S., Wyatt, A., Webb, J.K., O'Donnell, R., Mason, G., Rigby, M., Sirinathsighji, D., Hill, R.G., Rupniak, N.M.. Selective NMDA NR2B antagonists induce antinociception without motor dysfunction: correlation with restricted localisation of NR2B subunit in dorsal horn. *Neuropharmacology.* 1999, 38: 611-623.

[129] Qu, X.X., Cai, J., Li, M.J. Role of the spinal cord NR2Bcontaining NMDA receptors in the development of neuropathic pain. *Exp. Neurol.* 2009, 215: 298 –307.

[130] Woolf, C.J., Salter, M.W. Neuronal plasticity: increasing the gain in pain. *Science.* 2000, 288: 1765–1769.

[131] Malmberg, A.B., Chen, C., Tonegawa, S., Basbaum, A.I. Preserved acute pain and reduced neuropathic pain in mice lacking PKCgamma. *Science.* 1997, 278: 279-283.

[132] Brandt, M.R., Cummons, T.A., Potestio, L., Sukoff, S.J., Rosenzweig-Lipsonm S. Effects of the N-methyl-D-aspartate receptor antagonist perzinfotel [EAA-090; [2-(8,9-dioxo-2,6-diazabicyclo[5.2.0]non-1(7)-en-2-yl)-ethyl]phosphonic acid] on chemically induced thermal hypersensitivity. *J. Pharmacol. Exp. Ther.* 2005, 313:1379–1386.

[133] Hocking, G., Cousins, M.J. Ketamine in chronic pain management: an evidence-based review. *Anesth. Analg.* 2003, 97: 1730 –1739.

[134] Sang, C.N., Booher, S., Gilron, I., Parada, S., Max, M.B. Dextromethorphan and memantine in painful diabetic neuropathy and postherpetic neuralgia: efficacy and dose-response trials. *Anesthesiology* 2002, 96:1053–1061.

[135] Jackson KC. Pharmacotherapy for neuropathic pain. *Pain Pract.* 2006, (1): 27-33.

[136] Attal N, Mazaltarine G, Perrouin-Verbe B, Albert T; SOFMER French Society for Physical Medicine and Rehabilitation. Chronic neuropathic pain management in spinal cord injury patients. What is the efficacy of pharmacological treatments with a general mode of administration? (oral, transdermal, intravenous). *Ann Phys Rehabil Med.* 2009, Mar;52(2): 124-41.

[137] Rekand T1, Hagen EM, Grønning M. Chronic pain following spinal cord injury. *Tidsskr Nor Laegeforen*. 2012, 132(8): 974-9.

[138] Hwang JM, Wang CJ, Chou FP, Tseng TH, Hsieh YS, Hsu JD, Chu CY. Protective effect of baicalin on tert-butyl hydroperoxide-induced rat hepatotoxicity. *Arch Toxicol.* 2005, 79(2): 102-9.

[139] Li BQ, Fu T, Gong WH, Dunlop N, Kung H, Yan Y, Kang J, Wang JM. The flavonoid baicalin exhibits anti-inflammatory activity by binding to chemokines. *Immunopharmacology*. 2000, 49(3): 295-306.

[140] Jung SH, Kang KD, Ji D, Fawcett RJ, Safa R, Kamalden TA, Osborne NN. The flavonoid baicalin counteracts ischemic and oxidative insults to retinal cells and lipid peroxidation to brain membranes. *Neurochem Int.* 2008, 53(6-8): 325-37.

[141] Cao Y, Li G, Wang YF, Fan ZK, Yu DS, Wang ZD, Bi YL. Neuroprotective effect of baicalin on compression spinal cord injury in rats. *Brain Res*. 2010, 1357:115-23.

[142] Chou TC, Chang LP, Li CY, Wong CS, Yang SP. The antiinflammatory and analgesic effects of baicalin in carrageenan-evoked thermal hyperalgesia. *Anesth Analg*. 2003, 97(6): 1724-9.

[143] Cherng CH, Lee KC, Chien CC, Chou KY, Cheng YC, Hsin ST, Lee SO, Shen CH, Tsai RY, Wong CS. Baicalin ameliorates neuropathic pain by suppressing HDAC1 expression in the spinal cord of spinal nerve ligation rats. *J. Formos Med Assoc*. 2014, 113(8): 513-20.

[144] Fürst R, Zündorf I. Plant-Derived Anti-Inflammatory Compounds: Hopes and Disappointments regarding the Translation of Preclinical Knowledge into Clinical Progress. Mediators Inflamm. 2014, 2014:146832.

[145] Boots AW, Haenen GR, Bast A. Health effects of quercetin: from antioxidant to nutraceutical. *Eur J Pharmacol*. 2008, 585(2-3): 325-37.

[146] Hämäläinen M, Nieminen R, Vuorela P, Heinonen M, Moilanen E. Anti-inflammatory effects of flavonoids: genistein, kaempferol, quercetin, and daidzein inhibit STAT-1 and NF-kappaB activations, whereas flavone, isorhamnetin, naringenin, and pelargonidin inhibit only NF-kappaB activation along with their inhibitory effect on iNOS expression and NO production in activated macrophages. *Mediators Inflamm.* 2007, 2007:45673.

[147] Lee KW, Kang NJ, Heo YS, Rogozin EA, Pugliese A, Hwang MK, Bowden GT, Bode AM, Lee HJ, Dong Z. Raf and MEK protein kinases are direct molecular targets for the chemopreventive effect of quercetin, a major flavonol in red wine. *Cancer Res*. 2008, 68(3): 946-55.

[148] Dell'Agli M, Maschi O, Galli GV, Fagnani R, Dal Cero E, Caruso D, Bosisio E. Inhibition of platelet aggregation by olive oil phenols via cAMP-phosphodiesterase. *Br. J. Nutr.* 2008, 99(5): 945-51.

[149] Anjaneyulu M, Chopra K. Quercetin attenuates thermal hyperalgesia and cold allodynia in STZ-induced diabetic rats. *Indian J. Exp. Biol.* 2004, 42(8): 766-9.

[150] Schültke E, Griebel RW, Juurlink BH. Quercetin attenuates inflammatory processes after spinal cord injury in an animal model. *Spinal Cord.* 2010, 48(12): 857-61.

[151] Song Y, Liu J, Zhang F, Zhang J, Shi T, Zeng Z. Antioxidant effect of quercetin against acute spinal cord injury in rats and its correlation with the p38MAPK/iNOS signaling pathway. *Life Sci.* 2013, 92(24-26): 1215-21

[152] Schültke E, Kendall E, Kamencic H, Ghong Z, Griebel RW, Juurlink BH. Quercetin promotes functional recovery following acute spinal cord injury. *J. Neurotrauma.* 2003, 20(6): 583-91.

[153] Xu C, Xu W, Xu H, Xiong W, Gao Y, Li G, Liu S, Xie J, Tu G, Peng H, Qiu S, Liang S. Role of puerarin in the signalling of neuropathic pain mediated by P2X3 receptor of dorsal root ganglion neurons. *Brain Res Bull.* 2012, 87(1): 37-43.

[154] Meotti FC, Luiz AP, Pizzolatti MG, Kassuya CA, Calixto JB, Santos AR. Analysis of the antinociceptive effect of the flavonoid myricitrin: evidence for a role of the L-arginine-nitric oxide and protein kinase C pathways. *J. Pharmacol Exp Ther.* 2006, 316(2): 789-96.

[155] Meotti FC, Missau FC, Ferreira J, Pizzolatti MG, Mizuzaki C, Nogueira CW, Santos AR. Anti-allodynic property of flavonoid myricitrin in models of persistent inflammatory and neuropathic pain in mice. *Biochem Pharmacol.* 2006, 72(12): 1707-13.

[156] Meotti FC, Fachinetto R, Maffi LC, Missau FC, Pizzolatti MG, Rocha JB, Santos AR. Antinociceptive action of myricitrin: involvement of the K+ and Ca2+ channels. *Eur. J. Pharmacol.* 2007, 567(3): 198-205.

[157] Meotti FC, Posser T, Missau FC, Pizzolatti MG, Leal RB, Santos AR. Involvement of p38MAPK on the antinociceptive action of myricitrin in mice. *Biochem. Pharmacol.* 2007, 74(6): 924-31.

[158] Murakami A, Tanaka T, Lee JY, Surh YJ, Kim HW, Kawabata K, Nakamura Y, Jiwajinda S, Ohigashi H. Zerumbone, a sesquiterpene in subtropical ginger, suppresses skin tumor initiation and promotion stages in ICR mice. *Int. J. Cancer.* 2004, 110(4): 481-90.

[159] Betancur-Galvis LA, Morales GE, Forero JE, Roldan J. Cytotoxic and antiviral activities of Colombian medicinal plant extracts of the Euphorbia genus. *Mem Inst Oswaldo Cruz*. 2002, 97(4): 541-6.

[160] Dutra RC, Simão da Silva KA, Bento AF, Marcon R, Paszcuk AF, Meotti FC, Pianowski LF, Calixto JB. Euphol, a tetracyclic triterpene produces antinociceptive effects in inflammatory and neuropathic pain: the involvement of cannabinoid system. *Neuropharmacology*. 2012, 63(4): 593-605.

[161] Bernardes WA, Lucarini R, Tozatti MG, Flauzino LG, Souza MG, Turatti IC, Andrade e Silva ML, Martins CH, da Silva Filho AA, Cunha WR. Antibacterial activity of the essential oil from Rosmarinus officinalis and its major components against oral pathogens. *Z Naturforsch C*. 2010, 65(9-10): 588-93.

[162] Hudaib M, Speroni E, Di Pietra AM, Cavrini V. GC/MS evaluation of thyme (Thymus vulgaris L.) oil composition and variations during the vegetative cycle. *J. Pharm. Biomed Anal*. 2002, 29(4): 691-700.

[163] Jayaprakasha GK, Jagan Mohan Rao L, Sakariah KK. Volatile constituents from Cinnamomum zeylanicum fruit stalks and their antioxidant activities. *J. Agric. Food Chem*. 2003, 51(15): 4344-8.

[164] Mockute D, Bernotiene G, Judzentiene A. The essential oil of Origanum vulgare L. ssp. vulgare growing wild in vilnius district (Lithuania). *Phytochemistry*. 2001, 57(1): 65-9.

[165] Orav A, Stulova I, Kailas T, Müürisepp M. Effect of storage on the essential oil composition of Piper nigrum L. fruits of different ripening states. *J. Agric. Food Chem*. 2004, 52(9): 2582-6.

[166] Zheng GQ, Kenney PM, Lam LK. Sesquiterpenes from clove (Eugenia caryophyllata) as potential anticarcinogenic agents. *J. Nat. Prod.* 1992, 55(7): 999-1003.

[167] Gertsch J, Leonti M, Raduner S, Racz I, Chen JZ, Xie XQ, Altmann KH, Karsak M, Zimmer A. Beta-caryophyllene is a dietary cannabinoid. *Proc. Natl Acad Sci USA*. 2008, 105(26): 9099-104.

[168] Ghelardini C, Galeotti N, Di Cesare Mannelli L, Mazzanti G, Bartolini A. Local anaesthetic activity of beta-caryophyllene. *Farmaco*. 2001, 56(5-7):387-9.

[169] Legault J, Pichette A. Potentiating effect of beta-caryophyllene on anticancer activity of alpha-humulene, isocaryophyllene and paclitaxel. *J. Pharm. Pharmacol.* 2007, 59(12): 1643-7.

[170] Loizzo MR, Tundis R, Menichini F, Saab AM, Statti GA, Menichini F. Antiproliferative effects of essential oils and their major constituents in

human renal adenocarcinoma and amelanotic melanoma cells. *Cell Prolif.* 2008, 41(6): 1002-12.

[171] Calleja MA, Vieites JM, Montero-Meléndez T, Torres MI, Faus MJ, Gil A, Suárez A. The antioxidant effect of β-caryophyllene protects rat liver from carbon tetrachloride-induced fibrosis by inhibiting hepatic stellate cell activation. *Br. J. Nutr.* 2013, 109(3): 394-401.

[172] Galdino PM, Nascimento MV, Florentino IF, Lino RC, Fajemiroye JO, Chaibub BA, de Paula JR, de Lima TC, Costa EA. The anxiolytic-like effect of an essential oil derived from Spiranthera odoratissima A. St. Hil. leaves and its major component, β-caryophyllene, in male mice. *Prog Neuropsychopharmacol Biol. Psychiatry*. 2012, 38(2): 276-84.

[173] Klauke AL, Racz I, Pradier B, Markert A, Zimmer AM, Gertsch J, Zimmer A. The cannabinoid CB2 receptor-selective phytocannabinoid beta-caryophyllene exerts analgesic effects in mouse models of inflammatory and neuropathic pain. *Eur. Neuropsychopharmacol.* 2014, 24(4): 608-20.

[174] Otuki MF, Ferreira J, Lima FV, Meyre-Silva C, Malheiros A, Muller LA, Cani GS, Santos AR, Yunes RA, Calixto JB. Antinociceptive properties of mixture of alpha-amyrin and beta-amyrin triterpenes: evidence for participation of protein kinase C and protein kinase A pathways. *J. Pharmacol Exp. Ther.* 2005, 313(1): 310-8.

[175] Otuki MF, Vieira-Lima F, Malheiros A, Yunes RA, Calixto JB. Topical antiinflammatory effects of the ether extract from Protium kleinii and alpha-amyrin pentacyclic triterpene. *Eur. J. Pharmacol.* 2005, Jan 10;507(1-3): 253-9.

[176] Medeiros R, Otuki MF, Avellar MC, Calixto JB. Mechanisms underlying the inhibitory actions of the pentacyclic triterpene alpha-amyrin in the mouse skin inflammation induced by phorbol ester 12-O-tetradecanoylphorbol-13-acetate. *Eur. J. Pharmacol.* 2007, 559(2-3): 227-35.

[177] Vitor CE, Figueiredo CP, Hara DB, Bento AF, Mazzuco TL, Calixto JB. Therapeutic action and underlying mechanisms of a combination of two pentacyclic triterpenes, alpha- and beta-amyrin, in a mouse model of colitis. *Br. J. Pharmacol.* 2009, 157(6): 1034-44.

[178] da Silva KA, Paszcuk AF, Passos GF, Silva ES, Bento AF, Meotti FC, Calixto JB. Activation of cannabinoid receptors by the pentacyclic triterpene α,β-amyrin inhibits inflammatory and neuropathic persistent pain in mice. *Pain.* 2011, 152(8): 1872-87.

[179] Lin LZ, S. Yeh GA. Cordell, ni CZ, clardy J. Threeoxindole alkaloids from Gelsemium species. *Phytochemistry* 1991, 30: 679–683.

[180] Lin LZ, Hu SF, Cordell GA. 19 alpha-hydroxygelsamydinefrom Gelsemium elegans. *Phytochemistry* 1996, 43: 723–726.

[181] Liu M, Shen J, Liu H, Xu Y, Su YP, Yang J, Yu CX. Gelsenicine from Gelsemium elegans attenuates neuropathic and inflammatory pain in mice. *Biol Pharm Bull.* 2011, 34(12): 1877-80.

[182] Heubach JF, Schüle A. Cardiac effects of lappaconitine and N-deacetyllappaconitine, two diterpenoid alkaloids from plants of the Aconitum and Delphinium species. *Planta Med.* 1998, 64(1): 22-6.

[183] Liu JH, Zhu YX, Tang XC. Anti-inflammatory and analgesic activities of N-deacetyllappaconitine and lappaconitine. *Zhongguo Yao Li Xue Bao*. 1987, 8(4): 301-5.

[184] Shaheen F, Ahmad M, Khan MT, Jalil S, Ejaz A, Sultankhodjaev MN, Arfan M, Choudhary MI, Atta-ur-Rahman. Alkaloids of Aconitum laeve and their anti-inflammatory antioxidant and tyrosinase inhibition activities. *Phytochemistry*. 2005, 66(8): 935-40.

[185] Ono M, Satoh T. Pharmacological studies of lappaconitine. Analgesic activities. *Arzneimittelforschung*. 1988, 38(7): 892-5.

[186] Ou S, Zhao YD, Xiao Z, Wen HZ, Cui J, Ruan HZ. Effect of lappaconitine on neuropathic pain mediated by P2X3 receptor in rat dorsal root ganglion. *Neurochem Int*. 2011, 58(5): 564-73.

[187] Pivatto M, Antônio E. M. Crotti, Norberto P. Lopes, Ian Castro-Gamboa, Amanda de Rezende, Cláudio Viegas Jr., Maria Claudia M. Young, Maysa Furlan and Vanderlan S. Bolzani. Electrospray ionization mass spectrometry screening of piperidine alkaloids from Senna spectabilis (Fabaceae) extracts: fast identification of new constituents and co-metabolites. *J. Braz. Chem. Soc*. 16, 1431e1438.

[188] Alexandre-Moreira MS, Viegas C Jr, Palhares de Miranda AL, Bolzani Vda S, Barreiro EJ. Antinociceptive profile of (-)-spectaline: a piperidine alkaloid from Cassia leptophylla. *Planta Med.* 2003, 69(9): 795-9.

[189] da Silva KA, Manjavachi MN, Paszcuk AF, Pivatto M, Viegas C Jr, Bolzani VS, Calixto JB. Plant derived alkaloid (-)-cassine induces anti-inflammatory and anti-hyperalgesics effects in both acute and chronic inflammatory and neuropathic pain models. *Neuropharmacology*. 2012, 62(2): 967-77.

[190] Rice-Evans C. Plant polyphenols: free radical scavengers or chain-breaking antioxidants? *Biochem Soc Symp*. 1995, 61:103-16.

[191] Frei B, Higdon JV. Antioxidant activity of tea polyphenols in vivo: evidence from animal studies. *J. Nutr.* 2003, 133(10): 3275S-84S.

[192] Higdon JV, Frei B. Tea catechins and polyphenols: health effects, metabolism, and antioxidant functions. *Crit Rev Food Sci Nutr.* 2003, 43(1): 89-143.

[193] Nagle DG, Ferreira D, Zhou YD. Epigallocatechin-3-gallate (EGCG): chemical and biomedical perspectives. *Phytochemistry.* 2006, 67(17): 1849-55.

[194] Singh BN, Shankar S, Srivastava RK. Green tea catechin, epigallocatechin-3-gallate (EGCG): mechanisms, perspectives and clinical applications. *Biochem Pharmacol.* 2011, 82(12): 1807-21.

[195] Choi JI, Kim WM, Lee HG, Kim YO, Yoon MH. Role of neuronal nitric oxide synthase in the antiallodynic effects of intrathecal EGCG in a neuropathic pain rat model. *Neurosci Lett.* 2012, 510(1): 53-7.

[196] Kuang X, Huang Y, Gu HF, Zu XY, Zou WY, Song ZB, Guo QL. Effects of intrathecal epigallocatechin gallate, an inhibitor of Toll-like receptor 4, on chronic neuropathic pain in rats. *Eur. J. Pharmacol.* 2012, 676(1-3): 51-6.

[197] Renno WM, Al-Maghrebi M, Al-Banaw A. (-)-Epigallocatechin-3-gallate (EGCG) attenuates functional deficits and morphological alterations by diminishing apoptotic gene overexpression in skeletal muscles after sciatic nerve crush injury. *Naunyn Schmiedebergs Arch Pharmacol.* 2012, 385(8): 807-22.

[198] Khalatbary AR, Tiraihi T, Boroujeni MB, Ahmadvand H, Tavafi M, Tamjidipoor A. Effects of epigallocatechin gallate on tissue protection and functional recovery after contusive spinal cord injury in rats. *Brain Res.* 2010, 1306:168-75.

[199] Khalatbary AR, Ahmadvand H. Anti-inflammatory effect of the epigallocatechin gallate following spinal cord trauma in rat. *Iran Biomed J.* 2011, 15(1-2): 31-7.

[200] Renno WM, Al-Khaledi G, Mousa A, Karam SM, Abul H, Asfar S. (-)-Epigallocatechin-3-gallate (EGCG) modulates neurological function when intravenously infused in acute and, chronically injured spinal cord of adult rats. *Neuropharmacology.* 2014, 77:100-19.

[201] Yeh CW, Chen WJ, Chiang CT, Lin-Shiau SY, Lin JK. Suppression of fatty acid synthase in MCF-7 breast cancer cells by tea and tea polyphenols: a possible mechanism for their hypolipidemic effects. *Pharmacogenomics J.* 2003, 3(5): 267-76.

[202] Tian WX. Inhibition of fatty acid synthase by polyphenols. *Curr. Med. Chem.* 2006, 13(8): 967-77.

[203] Little JL, Kridel SJ. Fatty acid synthase activity in tumor cells. *Subcell Biochem*. 2008, 49:169-94.

[204] Linder ME, Deschenes RJ. Palmitoylation: policing protein stability and traffic. Nat Rev Mol Cell Biol. 2007, 8(1): 74-84.

[205] Nadolski MJ, Linder ME. Protein lipidation. *FEBS J.* 2007, 274(20): 5202-10.

[206] Ajuwon KM, Spurlock ME. Palmitate activates the NF-kappaB transcription factor and induces IL-6 and TNFalpha expression in 3T3-L1 adipocytes. *J. Nutr.* 2005, 135(8): 1841-6.

[207] Weigert C, Brodbeck K, Staiger H, Kausch C, Machicao F, Häring HU, Schleicher ED. Palmitate, but not unsaturated fatty acids, induces the expression of interleukin-6 in human myotubes through proteasome-dependent activation of nuclear factor-kappaB. *J. Biol Chem.* 2004, 279(23): 23942-52.

[208] Oberbach A, Schlichting N, Blüher M, Kovacs P, Till H, Stolzenburg JU, Neuhaus J. Palmitate induced IL-6 and MCP-1 expression in human bladder smooth muscle cells provides a link between diabetes and urinary tract infections. *PLoS One. 2010*, 5(5): e10882.

[209] Pan ZH, Segal MM, Lipton SA. Nitric oxide-related species inhibit evoked neurotransmission but enhance spontaneous miniature synaptic currents in central neuronal cultures. *Proc. Natl. Acad. Sci. USA*. 1996, 93(26): 15423-8.

[210] Saini R, Patel S, Saluja R, Sahasrabuddhe AA, Singh MP, Habib S, Bajpai VK, Dikshit M. Nitric oxide synthase localization in the rat neutrophils: immunocytochemical, molecular, and biochemical studies. *J. Leukoc Biol.* 2006, 79(3): 519-28.

[211] Tsang MY, Cowie SE, Rabkin SW. Palmitate increases nitric oxide synthase activity that is involved in palmitate-induced cell death in cardiomyocytes. *Nitric Oxide.* 2004, 10(1): 11-9.

[212] Qiu S, Li XY, Zhuo M. Post-translational modification of NMDA receptor GluN2B subunit and its roles in chronic pain and memory. *Semin Cell Dev Biol.* 2011, 22(5): 521-9.

[213] Demediuk P, Daly MP, Faden AI. Changes in free fatty acids, phospholipids, and cholesterol following impact injury to the rat spinal cord. *J. Neurosci Res*. 1989, 23(1): 95-106.

Index

A

B

C

F

G

H

I

J

K

N

O

P

T

U

V

W